Pharmacy Technician
Certification
Exam Review

Cheryl Aiken, PharmD, RPh
Formerly Director of Pharmacy Technology
Vermont Technical College
Randolph Center, Vermont

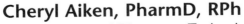

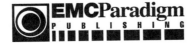

Senior Editor	Christine Hurney
Editorial Assistant	Susan Capecchi
Copy Editor	Ken Comer
Cover and Text Designer	Leslie Anderson
Desktop Production	Jack Ross
Proofreader	Jody McBride

Publishing Management Team

Bob Cassel, Publisher; Jeanne Allison, Senior Acquisitions Editor; Janice Johnson, Vice President of Marketing; Shelley Clubb, Electronic Design and Production Manager

---

Text and Encore CD ISBN 0-7638-2215-9
Product Number 01656
Text-only ISBN 0-7638-2216-7
Text-only Product Number 04656

© 2007 by Paradigm Publishing Inc.
    Published by EMC Corporation
    875 Montreal Way
    St. Paul, MN 55102
    (800) 535-6865
    E-mail: educate@emcp.com
    Web site: www.emcp.com

Printed in the United States of America.

10 9 8 7 6 5 4 3 2

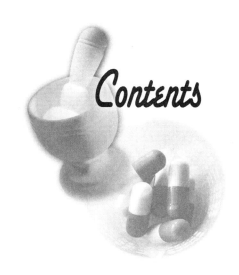

Contents

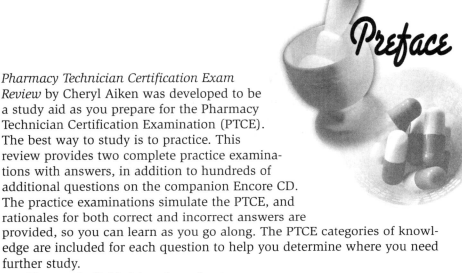
Preface

Pharmacy Technician Certification Exam Review by Cheryl Aiken was developed to be a study aid as you prepare for the Pharmacy Technician Certification Examination (PTCE). The best way to study is to practice. This review provides two complete practice examinations with answers, in addition to hundreds of additional questions on the companion Encore CD. The practice examinations simulate the PTCE, and rationales for both correct and incorrect answers are provided, so you can learn as you go along. The PTCE categories of knowledge are included for each question to help you determine where you need further study.

The text is divided into four chapters:

Chapter 1: Overview of Pharmacy Technician Certification Examination

Chapter 2: Preparing for the Pharmacy Technician Certification Examination

Chapter 3: First Practice Examination with answers and rationales

Chapter 4: Second Practice Examination with answers and rationales

KEY FEATURES

- Key concepts to focus study in preparation for PTCE
- Research-based test-taking strategies
- Examination overview
- Study strategies and PTCE categories
- Two model examinations written with the structure of and in the format of the PTCE
- Rationales for every answer

ALSO AVAILABLE

Encore CD that includes additional examination questions, a glossary and image bank for learning terminology, and interactive flash cards for learning the top prescribed drugs. The computerized text randomly selects questions to enable you to practice numerous times without repeating a test.

We wish you the best. Good luck!

REVIEWER

Jennifer Danielson, PharmD, RPh, MBA, CDE
Pikes Peak Community College
Colorado Springs, Colorado

ACKNOWLEDGMENTS

I would like to thank Mary Ann Stuhan, RPh, Cuyahoga Community College, for recommending that I write this book. A special thanks goes to Jennifer Danielson, PharmD, Pikes Peak Community College, for her advice and opinions about the text, and to Jeanne Allison and Christine Hurney at Paradigm Publishing for their help and patience. Finally, thank you to the love of my life, John L. Glick, for whose help and encouragement made this book possible.

—Cheryl Aiken

Overview of Pharmacy Technician Certification Examination

Learning Objectives

After completing this chapter, you should be able to:

- Understand the meaning of certification and recertification.
- Identify who should apply to take the examination.
- Explain how to apply to take the examination.
- List and describe the Pharmacy Technician Certification Examination content.

The Pharmacy Technician Certification Examination (PTCE) is the recognized test taken nationally by pharmacy technicians. The Pharmacy Technician Certification Board (PTCB) is a nongovernmental association responsible for the development and implementation of the rules and policies relating to national certification of pharmacy technicians. The primary goal of the PTCB is to enable pharmacy technicians to work effectively with pharmacists to provide patients with safe and effective pharmaceuticals.

MEANING OF CERTIFICATION AND RECERTIFICATION

Certification recognizes an individual for meeting predetermined qualifications in a specific area of study. Studying and passing the PTCE means the pharmacy technician meets the level of qualification for working in a pharmacy. Candidates passing the examination may use the designation certified pharmacy technician (CPhT) after their name. Although not required by all states to work in a pharmacy, many employers encourage certification among their technicians.

Recertification is the process of keeping your certification renewed. Every 2 years after you pass the PTCE, renewal of certification is required. During the 2-year period, a CPhT must earn 20 hours of pharmacy-related continuing education. This requirement also states that at least 1 hour of the continuing education must cover pharmacy law. Notification of recertification will arrive about 60 days before expiration of your old certification. Be sure to keep your address up to date with PTCB so your recertification packet arrives on time. Recertification, at present, costs $50.00, with an additional $15.00 if it is submitted during the 90-day late-fee period. If you recertify on-line, the recertification fee is $35.00 and may be paid with a credit card. Follow the directions carefully, otherwise a $10.00 reprocessing fee will be applied to returned applications.

WHO SHOULD APPLY?

Any person already working in a pharmacy should consider taking the certification examination. Additionally, individuals considering a career as a pharmacy technician should plan on studying and taking the PTCE. Many states reference the PTCE in their pharmacy rules and regulations and may require passing the certification examination before working as a pharmacy technician. Some employers encourage certification and include a monetary incentive for successful completion. Certification gives a sense of vocational identity to the pharmacy technician, as well as improving job satisfaction.

APPLYING FOR THE PHARMACY TECHNICIAN CERTIFICATION EXAMINATION

A visit to the PTCB's Web site (www.ptcb.org) will provide the prospective applicant with an abundance of information about the examination and an on-line application process. The examination is given three times a year across the United States with strict application submission dates. These are receipt deadlines and not postmark dates. You should check these dates for the next year and mark them on your calendar as a reminder to start the application process in time for the date you wish to take the examination. No part of your fee will be refunded unless you withdraw the application by the withdrawal deadline.

Overseas military technicians may sit for the PTCE during July and November using the DANTES Program. This information is available at the Web site.

ELIGIBILITY

Before sitting for the PTCE, the applicant must have a high school diploma or general education degree and not been convicted of a felony. Although a felony conviction does not absolutely bar you from taking the examination, each case will be evaluated individually. Include court documents or arrest reports related to the felony conviction by the application deadline. Anyone convicted of a drug or pharmacy-related felony will not be eligible to sit for the examination. You should also check with your state's board of pharmacy because a felony conviction may also prohibit registering with your state as a pharmacy technician.

APPLICATION PROCESS

You may apply either on-line or with a paper application. Do not do both. Follow the instructions carefully. Omissions of information, unsigned forms, or an incorrect payment will hold up your application process. All parts of the application need to be received by the deadline.

Your name on the application and admission ticket must match exactly the name on the valid government-issued photo identification (i.e., driver's license, military identification card, or passport). You will not be allowed to enter the examination and will forfeit your application fee if your identification is questionable.

Once you have filled in the application, sign and date your application. If your application is incomplete, you will be asked to resubmit your application and an additional $15.00 fee will be charged.

COST OF EXAMINATION

The application fee is $120.00. Pay with a certified check, money order, or corporate check. Personal checks, cash, or purchase orders will not be accepted. Credit card payments are also acceptable on the appropriate form or when applying on-line. Incomplete or inaccurate applications will be accessed an additional $15.00 fee.

Your admission ticket serves as your receipt. You will receive your ticket 3 weeks before the examination or it is available on-line in the same time period. Retain this ticket even after the examination as proof of payment.

EXAMINATION CONTENT

The examination contains 140 questions pertaining to activities performed by pharmacy technicians. The questions fall under three categories of training: (1) assisting the pharmacist in serving the patient, (2) maintaining medication and inventory management, and (3) participating in the administration and management of pharmacy practice. Table 1-1 lists the content of the PTCE.

Table 1-1 Contents of the Pharmacy Technician Certification Examination

Category I. Assisting the pharmacist in serving patients

1. Receive prescription or medication orders from the patient or patient's representative, prescriber, or other healthcare professional:
   - Accept new prescription or medication order from patient or patient's representative, prescriber, or other healthcare professional.
   - Accept new prescription or medication order electronically (e.g., by telephone, fax, or computer).
   - Accept refill request from patient or patient's representative, prescriber, or other healthcare professional.
   - Accept refill request electronically (e.g., by telephone, fax, or computer).
   - Contact prescriber-originator for clarification of prescription or medication order refill.
2. At the direction of the pharmacist, assist in obtaining from the patient or patient's representative such information as diagnosis or desired therapeutic outcome, medication use, allergies, adverse reactions, medical history and other relevant patient information, physical disability, and reimbursement mechanisms.
3. At the direction of the pharmacist, assist in obtaining from prescriber, other healthcare professionals, or the medical record such information as diagnosis or desired therapeutic outcome, medication use, allergies, adverse reactions, medical history and other relevant patient information, physical disability, and reimbursement mechanisms.
4. At the direction of the pharmacist, collect data (e.g., blood pressure, glucose) to assist the pharmacist in monitoring patient outcomes.
5. Assess prescription or medication order for completeness (e.g., patient's name and address), accuracy (e.g., consistency with products available), authenticity, legality, and reimbursement eligibility.
6. Update the medical record/patient profile with such information as medication history, allergies, medication duplication, as well as drug-disease, drug-drug, drug-laboratory, and drug-food interactions.
7. Process a prescription or medication order:
   - Enter prescription or medication order information onto patient profile.
   - Select the product or products for a generically written prescription or medication order.
   - Select the product or products for a brand-name prescription or medication order (consulting established formulary as appropriate).
   - Obtain medications or devices from inventory.
   - Measure, count, or calculate finished dose forms for dispensing.
   - Record preparation of prescription or medication, including any special requirements, for controlled substances.
   - Package finished dose forms (e.g., blister pack, vial).
   - Affix label and auxiliary label to container.
   - Assemble patient information materials.
   - Check for accuracy during processing of the prescription or medication order (e.g., matching National Drug Code [NDC] number).
   - Verify the measurements, preparation, and packaging of medications produced by other technicians.
   - Prepare prescription or medication order for final check by pharmacist.

Table 1-1 Contents of the Pharmacy Technician Certification
Examination—*continued*

Category I. Assisting the pharmacist in serving patients—*continued*

8. Compound a prescription or medication order:
   - Assemble equipment and supplies necessary for compounding the prescription or medication order.
   - Calibrate equipment (e.g., scale or balance, total parenteral nutrition [TPN] administration compounder) needed to compound the prescription or medication order.
   - Perform calculations required for usual dose determinations and preparation of compounded intravenous (IV) admixtures.
   - Compound medications (e.g., ointments, reconstituted antibiotic suspensions) for dispensing according to prescription formula or instructions.
   - Compound medications in anticipation of prescription or medication orders (e.g., bulk compounding for a specific patient).
   - Prepare sterile products (e.g., TPNs, piggybacks).
   - Prepare chemotherapy.
   - Record preparation and/or ingredients of medications (e.g., lot number, control number, expiration date).
9. Provision of medication to the patient or patient's representative:
   - Store medication before distribution.
   - Provide medication to patient or patient's representative.
   - Place medication in dispensing system (e.g., unit dose cart, robotics).
   - Deliver medication to patient-care unit.
   - Record distribution of prescription medication.
   - Record distribution of controlled substances.
   - Record distribution of investigational drugs.
10. Determine charges and obtain reimbursement for services.
11. Communicate with third-party payers to determine or verify coverage and obtain prior authorizations.
12. Provide supplemental information (e.g., patient package leaflets, computer-generated information, videos) as requested or required.
13. Ask patient whether counseling by pharmacist is desired.
14. Perform drug administration functions under appropriate supervision (e.g., perform drug or IV rounds, anticipate refill of drugs or IVs).
15. Assist the pharmacist in monitoring patient laboratory values (e.g., blood pressure, cholesterol values).

Category II. Maintaining medication and inventory control systems

1. Identify pharmaceuticals, durable medical equipment, devices, and supplies to be ordered (e.g., want book).
2. Place orders for pharmaceuticals, durable medical equipment, devices, and supplies (including investigational and hazardous products and devices), and expedite emergency orders in compliance with legal, regulatory, professional, and manufacturers' requirements.
3. Receive goods and verify against specifications on original purchase orders.
4. Place pharmaceuticals, durable medical equipment, devices, and supplies (including hazardous materials and investigational products) in inventory under proper storage conditions.

Continues

Table 1-1 Contents of the Pharmacy Technician Certification Examination—*continued*

Category II. Maintaining medication and inventory control systems—*continued*

5. Perform nonpatient-specific distribution of pharmaceuticals, durable medical equipment, devices, and supplies (e.g., crash carts, nursing station stock, automated dispensing systems).
6. Remove from inventory expired, discontinued, and slow-moving pharmaceuticals; durable medical equipment; devices; and supplies.
7. Remove from inventory recalled pharmaceuticals, durable medical equipment, devices, and supplies.
8. Communicate changes in product availability (e.g., formulary changes, recalls) to pharmacy staff, patient or patient's representative, physicians, and other healthcare professionals.
9. Implement and monitor policies and procedures to deter theft and drug diversion.
10. Maintain a record of controlled substances received, stored, and removed from inventory.
11. Perform required inventories and maintain associated records.
12. Maintain record-keeping systems for repackaging, bulk compounding, recalls, and returns of pharmaceuticals, durable medical equipment, devices, and supplies.
13. Compound medications in anticipation of prescription or medication orders (e.g., bulk compounding).
14. Perform quality assurance (QA) tests on compounded medications (e.g., for bacterial growth; for sodium, potassium, dextrose levels; for radioactivity).
15. Repackage finished dose forms for dispensing.
16. Participate in QA programs related to products or supplies, or both (e.g., formulary revision, nursing unit audits, performance evaluations of wholesalers).
17. Communicate with representatives of pharmaceutical and equipment suppliers.

Category III. Participating in the administration and management of pharmacy practice

1. Coordinate written, electronic, and oral communications throughout the practice setting (e.g., route phone calls, faxes, verbal and written refill authorizations), and disseminate policy changes.
2. Update and maintain information (e.g., insurance information, patient demographics, provider information, reference material).
3. Collect productivity information (e.g., the number of prescriptions filled, fill times, money collected, rejected claim status).
4. Participate in quality improvement activities (e.g., medication error reports, customer satisfaction surveys, delivery audits, internal audits of processes).
5. Generate QA reports.
6. Implement and monitor the practice setting for compliance with federal, state, and local laws, regulations, and professional standards (e.g., materials safety data sheet [MSDS], eyewash centers, Joint Commission on Accreditation of Healthcare Organizations [JCAHO] standards).
7. Implement and monitor policies and procedures for sanitation management, handling of hazardous waste (e.g., needles), and infection control (e.g., protective clothing, laminar flow hood, other equipment cleaning).

Table 1-1 Contents of the Pharmacy Technician Certification Examination—*continued*

Category III. Participating in the administration and management of pharmacy practice—continued
8. Perform and record routine sanitation, maintenance, and calibration of equipment (e.g., automated dispensing equipment, balances, robotics, refrigerator temperatures).
9. Maintain and use manual or computer-based information systems to perform job-related activities (e.g., update prices, generate reports and labels, perform utilization tracking and inventory).
10. Maintain software for automated dispensing technology, including point-of-care drug dispensing cabinets.
11. Perform billing and accounting functions (e.g., personal charge accounts, third-party rejections, third-party reconciliation, census maintenance, prior authorization).
12. Communicate with third-party payers to determine or verify coverage.
13. Conduct staff training.
14. Aid in establishing, implementing, and monitoring policies and procedures.

Source: Pharmacy Technician Certification Board, www.ptcb.org/exam/content.asp (accessed October 11, 2005). Used with permission.

Category I. Assisting the Pharmacist in Serving the Patient

This area is the major portion of the examination. Sixty-four percent of your knowledge is tested in this area. When studying for this part, remember that you demonstrate some of these skills every day at work. Given that this test includes knowledge on both community and institutional pharmacy, you will need to spend more time studying the area in which you do not work on a daily basis.

Some areas you will want to make sure you know are:
Community Pharmacy Knowledge Areas
Federal laws, regulations, codes of ethics and standards related to pharmacy practice
Abbreviations and terminology
Generic and brand names of pharmaceuticals
Strength and dose, dose forms, physical appearance, route of administration, and duration of drug therapy
Effects of a patient's age and disabilities on drug therapy
Drug information resources, both printed and electronic
Drug indications
Practice site policies and procedures
Information to be obtained from the patient or patient's representative
Requirements for prescription refills
Verification of U.S. Drug Enforcement Administration (DEA) numbers

Techniques for detecting forged or altered prescriptions
Techniques for detecting medication errors
Equipment and supplies for drug administration
Nonprescription drug products
Monitoring and screening equipment
Medical and surgical supplies
Proper storage conditions
Automated dispensing technology
Packaging requirements
Components of NDC number
Purpose of lot and expiration dates
Prescription label information
Auxiliary label requirements
Requirements for patient package inserts
Special directions and precautions
Assessing compliance
Action to take for a missed dose
Medication mailing requirements
Requirements for controlled substances
Dispensing record keeping requirements
Pharmacy calculations and measurement systems
Extemporaneous compounding of oral dosage forms, sterile noninjectable products and nonsterile products
Controlled substance documentation
Use of computers in pharmacy practice
Backup manual system for power failures
Customer service skills
Confidentiality requirements
Legal counseling requirements

Institutional Pharmacy or Home Infusion Pharmacy Knowledge

Federal regulations, codes of ethics, and standards
Abbreviations and terminology
Generic and brand names of pharmaceuticals
Strength and dose, dose forms, physical appearance, route of administration, and duration of drug therapy
The effects of a patient's age and disabilities on drug therapy
Drug information resources, both printed and electronic
Drug indications
Practice site policies and procedures
Techniques for detecting medication errors
Equipment and supplies for drug administration
Nonprescription drug products
Medical and surgical supplies

Proper storage conditions
Automated dispensing technology
Packaging and repackaging requirements
Components of NDC number
Purpose of lot and expiration dates

Information on medication order label
Special directions and precautions for patient representative
Action to be taken in case of missed dose
Delivery systems for distributing medication
Controlled substance dispensing
Investigational drug dispensing
Record-keeping requirements
Automatic stop orders
Restricted medication orders
Quality Improvement methods
Pharmacy calculations and measurement systems
Drug stability
Incompatibilities
Equipment calibration techniques
Procedures for preparing IV admixtures and TPN
Procedure for preparing chemotherapy
Aseptic technique and USP 797
Extemporaneous compounding
Infection control procedures
Requirements for handling hazardous waste
Customer service techniques
Communication techniques
Confidentiality requirements
Use of computers in pharmacy practice

Other Areas of Knowledge

Preparation of radiopharmaceuticals
Therapeutic equivalence
Epidemiology
Risk factors for disease
Anatomy and physiology
Signs and symptoms of disease states
Standard and abnormal laboratory values
Drug interactions
Pharmacology (i.e., mechanism of action)
Common side effect and adverse effects, allergies, and contraindications
Role of nondrug therapy
Cash handling and reimbursement

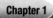

Category II. Maintaining Medication and Inventory Control Systems

Although this area represents only 25% of the total examination's content, it is an important area of knowledge for the technician as they do most of the ordering, receiving, and inventory management. You demonstrate many of these skills every day but should review the knowledge requirements and spend time studying areas about which you feel less knowledgeable.

Areas of Knowledge

Laws and regulations related to obtaining medications and supplies
Drug testing, approval, and removal for market
Purchasing policies and practices
Dose forms and routes of administration
Formulary or approved stock lists
Reordering and drug usage
Inventory receiving procedures
Bioavailability standards for generic substitution
DEA order forms
Record keeping for repackaging, recalls, and refunded products
Inventory systems
Products used in packaging and repackaging
Risk management opportunities
U.S. Food and Drug Administration (FDA) recall classifications
Returning expired or unsaleable products
Disposal of products
Professional standards for operating a pharmacy
Laws and regulations on obtaining, labeling, dispensing, distributing, and administering medications
Various practice setting medication distribution
Compounded medication preparation, storage, and documentation
Preparation of medication in anticipation of prescription of medication order
Storage and handling of hazardous materials and waste, including MSDS information
Medication distribution requirements for controlled substances, investigation drugs, and hazardous materials
Communication channels for followup and problem resolution
QA practices for medication and inventory systems

Category III. Participating in the Administration and Management of Pharmacy Practice

Eleven percent of the examination focuses on this area of pharmacy practice for technicians. Many technicians have little experience in this area.

Knowledge in this area will not only help make your pharmacy run better, but will also give the technician an increased sense of job satisfaction. Understanding why a specific task must be done makes even the most mundane chore, such as checking refrigerator temperature, take on a new meaning of importance. Study in this area might include talking to the pharmacy manager, director of pharmacy at a hospital, or district manager.

Areas of Knowledge

Mission statements, goals, and objectives; organizational structure; and policy and procedures

Channels of communication in an organization

Resource allocations

Measures of productivity, efficiency, and customer satisfaction

Written, oral, and electronic forms of communication

Required operational licenses and certificates

Roles and responsibilities of pharmacy personnel

Legal and regulatory requirements for the pharmacy (i.e., counters, equipment, references, storage)

Professional standards for accreditation

Quality improvement standards and guidelines

State board regulations (Although exact content is not tested, knowing who has regulatory authority is important.)

Storage requirement for equipment and supplies

Hazardous substances storage, handling, and disposal

Treatment of exposure to hazardous substances

Security system for pharmacy staff, customers, and property

Laminar flow hood maintenance

Infection control

Sanitation requirements

Equipment maintenance and calibration procedures

Supply procurement procedures

Technology used in all pharmacy situations

Equipment purpose and function

Documentation required for sanitation, maintenance, and equipment calibration

Americans with Disabilities Act requirements

Manual and computer based pharmacy systems

Security of data

Downtime emergency procedure

Safe storage of data

Legal requirements of archiving data

Third-party reimbursement systems

Healthcare reimbursement systems

Billing and accounting procedure

Information sources for quality improvement data
Documentation of medication errors, adverse drug reactions, and
  product integrity
Staff training techniques
Employee performance evaluation and feedback

You must be familiar with over 100 knowledge areas. Although this task
may appear overwhelming, you will already be knowledgeable about many
areas and can focus studying on areas of less familiarity. Pharmacy is an
expansive and dynamic field, and you cannot know everything, but you
should have a well-rounded knowledge base.

Preparing for the Pharmacy Technician Certification Examination

Learning Objectives

After completing this chapter, you should be able to:

- List all the items to bring to the examination.
- Make a plan for studying for the examination.
- Describe techniques for how to take a multiple-choice examination.
- Explain how the examination is scored.
- Explain when the score is reported.
- Explain the process for hand scoring.

ITEMS TO BRING TO THE EXAMINATION

On the day of the examination, you need to arrive at the testing site between 7:30 and 8:00 in the morning. If you are unfamiliar with the route you will be traveling to take the test, leave yourself extra time, or plan on arriving the night before and staying with friends or in a comfortable accommodation.

You need to bring a few items with you to be admitted to the examination site. An admission ticket should have been sent to you approximately 3 weeks before the examination, or you should have printed one from the Pharmacy Technician Certification Board (PTCB) Internet site. You must have this admission ticket.

Identification is required for entrance. Bring a valid government picture identification, such as a passport, driver's license with photograph, or U.S. Armed Forces photo identification. The document should be clean and clear and not be taped. Your name must appear exactly as it appears on your admission ticket. If your name or social security number does not match, you will not be permitted to take the examination. If you forget this document, you will not be able to take the examination.

You should bring several No. 2 pencils with erasers and a hand-held, nonprogrammable, nonprinting calculator that is battery or solar powered. Do not bring a scientific calculator or a calculator that performs fractions; they will not be allowed in the examination room.

Reference materials, books, or papers are not allowed in the examination room. Your test booklet will serve as your scratch paper. Cellular phones, pagers, or other electronic devices are not permitted in the examination room, either. Leave these items in your car or at home.

No questions about the examination's content may be asked during the testing time. Written comments about the accuracy or content of any questions may be made on the available forms. The PTCB Certification Council will review these comments. Do not expect an individual response. If you have any comment about the testing facility, test supervision, or a related matter, contact Professional Examination Services (PES), 475 Riverside Drive, New York, NY 10115, FAX: (212) 367-4343, within 2 weeks of the day of the examination. The PTCB hires this company to administer the examination across the country.

Items to Bring to the Examination

- Admission ticket
- Valid photo identification
- Several No. 2 pencils
- Erasers
- Nonprogrammable calculator

STUDYING FOR THE EXAMINATION

1. Know the material on which you will be tested. Review test outlines if available. The Pharmacy Technician Certification Examination (PTCE) has 140 multiple-choice questions. Each question has four choices, with only one answer being the correct or best answer. Fifteen of these questions will not count toward your final grade. These questions are used to provide statistical information for the content of future examinations. They are randomly placed throughout the examination and not identified. The other 125 questions will test on the knowledge and responsibilities of the pharmacy technician in the three function areas as discussed in Chapter 1 of this review book or on the PTCB Web site. These questions are randomly placed throughout the examination. You will be given 3 hours to complete the examination. Do not plan on staying at the examination site later than 12:00 P.M.

2. Study all key topics that will appear on the examination. Any time spent studying is time well spent. Whether you are reviewing material for a project at work or taking the examination as a lifelong learner, you will find that this knowledge and testing provides you with greater satisfaction at your job and in your life. Although there are no guarantees that study-

ing hard gets you a passing grade, the odds are better if you do put the time into the effort. Because of the number of questions being asked on the PTCE, you must know a broad range of material. Chapter 1 in this book lists most of the knowledge areas with which you should be familiar to pass the examination. Once you feel comfortable with the information, or if you are unsure where your weaknesses are, take a practice examination, such as the practice examinations in this book. No more than 3 hours should be taken to complete the examination. Once completed, compare your answers to the answers provided.

Studying for a multiple-choice examination is different from other types of examinations. You are not being asked to pull the correct answer entirely from memory. The answer is on the page. Even a lucky guess gets points.

3. Spread out your review over a period of weeks. Focused reviews over time are more effective than cramming. Cramming for examinations never works. You will be using this information for years to come, not just learning for one test and forgetting it. By starting early in your review and spending a little time every week, your knowledge and skills will grow. Invite other pharmacy technicians to join a study group. Contact your local chapter of the American Association of Pharmacy Technicians or National Association of Pharmacy Technicians and inquire about the examination. Pick the brains of pharmacy technicians who have already taken and passed the examination. Ask for help in understanding concepts from your peers and the pharmacy staff. Calculations are always a difficult area to study; ask pharmacists to spend some time explaining how to perform calculations. By starting early, others will be more willing to help you study. Remember, getting a good night's sleep the night before a major examination is better than staying up late studying. Your mind will be clearer, and you will make better choices.

4. Outline your text, and mark topics that need a more concentrated review. When you use review books, mark them up. Highlight and underline areas that you want to be able to find again. Highlight the questions you answer incorrectly on the practice examinations, and review information relating to them. Write yourself cheat sheets or flash cards to carry around with you to study when you have a few minutes.

5. Try to predict questions that may be on the test, and then test your skills in answering them. Although none of us knows for certain what will be on the examination, certain areas of knowledge are always tested. An important point to remember is that numerous versions of the test are distributed in the examination room at one time. Your neighbor will not

necessarily have the same test as you do. The grading process is discussed later in this chapter.

6. If possible, study in the room where the test will be given. Although doing so may not be possible for most of the applicants, if you arrive early to familiarize with the space before the examination, you will find you are less nervous. Running in at the last minute is not the ideal way to prepare for starting an examination. If circumstances do make you short on time, do not panic, take a deep breath, and try to relax. Then start the examination.

For example, a recent graduate of a pharmacy technician program showed up at the site that she was told the examination would be given. She arrived early, had a good night's sleep, and brought all the items she needed with her only to find the examination site had been moved. The new testing site was across town in an area with which she was unfamiliar. She was a few minutes late, but the instructors, after hearing her story, allowed her to enter and take the examination. Afterwards, she was sure she had failed just because of the mix-up. As the story turned out, she passed and has been an excellent pharmacy technician ever since. The moral of the story: have faith in yourself even under the worst of circumstances.

On the Day of the Test

- Get enough sleep the night before the test. Also make sure you have gotten adequate sleep the week before the test.
- Arrive at the testing location early, and choose a comfortable working area.
- Dress casually and comfortably. Take extra time planning appropriate clothes.
- Arrive prepared with necessary supplies.
- Do a relaxation exercise, such as deep breathing, before the test.

TIPS FOR MULTIPLE-CHOICE QUESTIONS

1. Plan your time. You have 3 hours to complete the examination. Do not get stuck on one question and not leave time to finish the examination. If you are not sure of the answer to the question within 30 to 60 seconds, move on and come back later.

2. Read the whole item. Identify what the question is asking. Take the item at face value, and do not read too much into the question. Do not waste time looking for tricks; they usually do not exist. Try reading the question with all the possible answers, and it may jog your memory.

3. Remember that only one preferred answer exists even though more than one answer might appear to be correct. When writing multiple-choice questions, one correct answer and three distracters are assigned. The distracters are usually terms or work you know, but only if you studied the information do you understand their significance. In calculation questions, distracters will use the numbers in various wrong ways to get answers that you might get if you are not sure how to do the calculations. You might try covering up the answers and try to anticipate the correct answer before you are distracted by the given choices. For calculations, do not look at the answers. Solve the problem, then check if any of the answers match your answer.

4. Use the process of elimination when you do not know the answer. Eliminate the most obviously wrong answer first, then the second, and then make your best decision between the last two choices. This tactic gives you a 50% chance of getting the answer right. Ignore the people who tell you to look for patterns in the answers. Tests are usually written with the answers randomly placed, and the authors do not view the answer sheet for patterns.

As You Take the Test

- Listen, read, and follow the directions carefully.
- Make sure to fill out the answer sheet correctly.
- Look over the test before answering any questions. Scanning the test will provide you with key information about the scope and difficulty of the test.
- First answer the questions that are easiest for you.
- Answer the questions in order but postpone questions that challenge you until later in the test.
- On your second pass through the test, ignore the answered questions and focus only on the questions you did not answer.
- Never leave a question unanswered; no penalty is given for guessing. (Time management is key; answering all the items on the test is to your advantage.)
- Change your answers only when you are certain that you made a mistake. Your first answer is usually the correct one.

5. If you are still unsure about which answer is correct, select the longer or more descriptive answer of the remaining answer set, although a good author will write all answers to a similar length.

6. If the answer set presents a range of numbers, eliminate the highest and lowest, and then select from the middle range of numbers.

7. Slow down when you see negative words in the question. Look for words such as *not* or *except*. In this case, you need to identify the false statement instead of the true statement. Read the question carefully, and underline the negative word to remind yourself. Make sure you understand what the question is asking you.

8. Items that contain "absolutes" such as *always, never, must, all,* and *none* severely limit the meaning of the item. Statements that contain absolutes are usually incorrect.

9. Be sure to fill in the answer sheet correctly. If you erase, make sure you erase completely. Do not leave any stray pencil marks on your answer sheet that the computer might be read incorrectly. Do not be in a hurry to start, thereby forgetting to fill in your name and identification information. Having a passing test with no name on it would be a shame.

10. If you feel a question on the exam is ambiguous, deficient in accuracy or content, or misleading, be sure to fill out the form provided at the conclusion of the exam to report such questions. All comments about questions will be reviewed by the PTCB Certification Council.

SCORING THE EXAMINATION

The scoring of the PTCE is probably different from any other test you have ever taken. The passing score is not a specific number of questions right because of the variation in the difficulty of the questions that make up the different examinations. One examination may be slightly easier or more difficult than another. In one sense, the difference is similar to comparing apples and oranges. For this reason, the questions in the examination are weighted differently, based on their level of difficulty. Once this process is complete, the weighted grades are converted to the score that is reported. This factor allows the test to reflect the level of ability of each individual regardless of which examination form is taken. A score of at least 650 is necessary to pass the examination. Total scores may range between 300 and 900.

During the grading process, the PTCB takes ambiguous test items into consideration. The item may be scored with more than one correct answer with no penalty to the candidate. The investigation into the question may be to your favor and boost your grade if the question is determined to be ambiguous. This demonstrates the importance of filling out the form for questions you believe are misleading or deficient in accuracy or content.

The answer sheets are scored electronically. The answers are stored in a database from which scored reports will eventually be generated. The PTCB goes to great length to ensure quality in the process. A preliminary report of the test items is reviewed by the PTCB Certification Council to make sure the questions test as expected. This procedure allows for adjustment of flawed test items. Once this task is accomplished, all the answer sheets are scored again with the new scoring key. The resulting score is your final report. The passing score is based on the total score for all questions. You do not have to receive a passing score in each of the three functions test.

REPORTING SCORES

Professional Examination Service (PES) will mail your score report to the address on file in approximately 30 days after the examination date. During this same period, a pass-fail grade is available at the PTCB Web site. Neither PTCB nor PES will disclose scores over the telephone, by FAX, or e-mail. For candidates who do not receive a score within 60 days of the examination date, contact PES in writing at 475 Riverside Drive, New York, NY 10115, and a duplicate score report will be issued at no cost. If you wait more than 90 days from the examination date, PES will require a $15.00 processing fee. Individual test scores are only released to the candidate.

The scored report mailed to the candidate will provide a breakdown of performance in the three function areas, which will provide valuable information on the candidate's weaknesses and strengths in the three different areas. This information is intended for the candidate only, and passing is based on the total score of all three areas.

REQUESTING HAND SCORING OF THE ANSWER SHEET

If you receive a failing grade on the PTCE, you may request that your answer sheet be scored by hand. This request must be made in writing to PES within 90 days of the date of the examination. Your request must include your social security number, test date, and signature. A *Request for Hand Scoring of Answer Sheet* is available at the PTCB Web site. A charge of $50.00 must be included with your request as a certified check or money order payable to Professional Examination Service. Do not request hand scoring until you have received your score report from PES. Hand scoring results are final, and you will be notified of any change in your score.

REEXAMINATION

If you do not receive a passing score on your examination, eligible candidates may take the examination as many times as necessary to earn a passing grade. A new application with appropriate documentation and application fee must be submitted each time.

Chapter 2

RECOGNITION OF CERTIFICATION

You passed your examination. Now what? First of all, congratulations. Start using the designation Certified Pharmacy Technician (CPhT) after your name. You have demonstrated your knowledge of the skills necessary to work as a pharmacy technician. You will soon receive a certificate for framing and a wallet card. Your certification is valid for 2 years. During that time, you need to continue to update your knowledge by attending continuing education programs, reading pharmacy related journals, and submitting the appropriate paperwork for credit. You need 20 hours of continuing education every 2 years to apply for recertification.

REVOCATION OF CERTIFICATION

This certificate is important and imparts a vocational identity to the job you perform as a pharmacy technician. A significant number of reasons can lead to the revocation of your certification. *Your Guidebook to PTCB Certification* contains this information. In particular, being convicted of a felony or a crime involving moral turpitude (including the illegal sale, distribution, or use of controlled substances and other prescription drugs) or making false statements in connection with certification or recertification may cause your certification to be revoked. Refer to your guide for more information.

Disclaimer
All the information provided in this section is also available and, in some cases, in more depth in the *Your Guidebook to PTCB Certification* or at the PTCB Web site (www.ptcb.org). Always refer to these resources for the exact requirements and fee schedules for the PTCE.

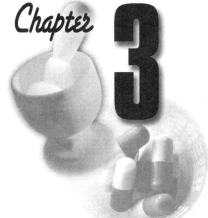

Chapter 3

First Practice Examination

This test contains 140 multiple-choice questions. Read the questions and select the best answer for each question.

1. Which of the following drugs may cause photosensitivity?
   a. phenytoin
   b. famotidine
   c. tetracycline
   d. levothyroxine

2. The cost of 1000 capsules of amoxicillin is $27.95. How much will you have to charge a customer for 30 capsules to yield a 34% margin?
   a. $8.39
   b. $0.84
   c. $1.13
   d. $9.50

3. How many grams of 5% hydrocortisone ointment can be made with 10 g of hydrocortisone powder?
   a. 200 g
   b. 2000 g
   c. 0.5 g
   d. 50 g

4. How many 30 mg lansoprazole capsules will you need to make a 2-week supply of lansoprazole oral solution for a patient who must take 30 mg per nasogastric (NG) tube bid?
   a. 14 capsules
   b. 28 capsules
   c. 30 capsules
   d. 840 capsules

5. Which medication listed does *not* have to be dispensed in a child-resistant container?
   a. oxycodone 5 mg tablets
   b. levofloxacin 500 mg tablets
   c. digoxin 0.125 mg tablets
   d. pancrelipase capsules

6. The dispensing fee for prescriptions is $6.50. How much should you charge for 50 tablets of amitriptyline 25 mg if 100 tablets cost the pharmacy $12.43?
   a. $12.72
   b. $9.47
   c. $7.12
   d. $6.22

7. Mrs. Jones asked you to refill her heart medication. Which of the following medications on her profile will you refill?
   a. Nexium
   b. Cardizem
   c. Premarin
   d. Zoloft

Chapter 3

8. How many grams of dextrose are needed to compound 250 mL of a 45% dextrose solution?
   a. 45 g
   b. 112.5 g
   c. 11.25 g
   d. 11,250 g

9. Aseptic technique is the process of manipulating sterile products to prevent
   a. introduction of an active ingredient.
   b. introduction of pathogens.
   c. introduction of water.
   d. introduction of sepsis.

10. You purchase 10 cases of diaper rash cream with a manufacturer's discount of 15% if the invoice is paid in full within 30 days. The full price is $25.00 a case. What is the price for all 10 cases if paid in full before the 30 days pass?
    a. $21.25
    b. $250.00
    c. $37.50
    d. $212.50

11. How many 80 mg doses of gentamicin can be made from a multidose vial with 20 mL of a 40 mg/mL gentamicin solution?
    a. 10 doses
    b. 0.5 dose
    c. 40 doses
    d. 100 doses

12. Which of the following drugs is a schedule I controlled substance?
    a. methadone
    b. codeine
    c. opium
    d. heroin

13. How much epinephrine is in 10 mL of a 1:10,000 solution?
    a. 1 mg
    b. 1 g
    c. 0.1 mg
    d. 0.01 g

14. To prepare a medication order for 0.225% sodium chloride solution, the pharmacy technician will mix the stock solutions 0.9% sodium chloride and sterile water in which ratio?
    a. 1:1
    b. 1:2
    c. 1:3
    d. 1:4

Chapter 3

15. The name for the official list of medications approved for use in an institution is called a
    a. United States Pharmacopeia.
    b. care plan.
    c. *Orange Book.*
    d. formulary.

16. A prescription with the directions "2 tablets stat 1 po daily × 4 for URI" would be dispensed with which of the following directions?
    a. Take two tablets now then one tablet by mouth daily for 4 days for urinary tract infection.
    b. Take two tablets now then one tablet by mouth daily for 4 days for upper respiratory infection.
    c. Take two now then one daily for 4 days for upper respiratory infection.
    d. Take two tablets as soon as possible then one tablet daily for upper respiratory infection.

17. Where should hazardous substances needing refrigeration be stored?
    a. next to other refrigerated products on wire racks
    b. separate from other drugs in bins that prevent breakage and control leakage
    c. in the hood where chemotherapy is admixed
    d. at room temperature as long as the room is air conditioned

18. For a generic drug to be considered bioequivalent, it must contain the same active ingredient as does the original, as well as be identical in strength, route of administration, and
    a. color.
    b. inactive ingredients.
    c. price.
    d. dose form.

19. The pharmacy technician receives a prescription for Tiazac, and a review of the patient's profile reveals a prescription for verapamil, which was filled a week ago. What should the pharmacy technician do?
    a. Fill the prescription because it is not for the same drug.
    b. Notify the pharmacist of a potential duplication of therapy.
    c. Call the physician to discuss the duplication of therapy.
    d. Discontinue the verapamil prescription and fill the Tiazac.

20. Which of the following concepts does the federal law OBRA-90 require?
    a. confidentiality
    b. compliance
    c. medication errors
    d. counseling

21. The pharmacy and therapeutics (P&T) committee's primary function is to
    a. formulate policies pertaining to pharmaceutical use in the hospital.
    b. establish job descriptions for hospital employees.
    c. review investigation drug research and publish articles.
    d. establish care plans for the treatment of disease states.

22. A Pyxis machine is an example of a(n)
    a. pneumatic delivery system.
    b. class-100 environment.
    c. automatic dispensing technology.
    d. sterile compounding machine.

23. Where is the volume of fluid measured in a conical graduate?
    a. top of the meniscus
    b. center of the meniscus
    c. bottom of the meniscus
    d. one mark above the bottom of the meniscus

24. A medication order for ampicillin 1 g IVPB q4h is started at 6:00 A.M. When will the next two doses be given?
    a. 1200, 1800
    b. 1000, 1400
    c. 0900, 1300
    d. 0800, 1200

25. How many milligrams are in a ¼ gr thyroid USP tablet?
    a. 15 mg
    b. 25 mg
    c. 30 mg
    d. 60 mg

26. A pharmacy technician receives a class-II drug recall from the manufacturer. What should he or she do?
    a. Call all patients who have received the drug in the last year, and have them return it to the pharmacy.
    b. File the recall, and wait until you receive notice from the wholesaler.
    c. Check the inventory for the recalled lots, and send any recalled drug back to the manufacturer.
    d. Post the recall on the announcement board in case anyone is interested.

27. The reason a Coumadin drug utilization evaluation (DUE) might be done is because it is a medicine with a high
    a. rate of side effects and drug interactions.
    b. cost index and a low margin.
    c. incidence of patients sharing prescriptions.
    d. incidence of addiction and abuse potential.

28. Which of the following intravenous (IV) antibiotics is an antineoplastic and should a nurse never mix on the patient unit?
    a. erythromycin
    b. gentamicin
    c. azithromycin
    d. bleomycin

Chapter 3

29. You are asked to compound a pediatric suspension of spironolactone that is 1 mg/5 mL. The prescription is for a 30-day supply, and the patient takes 1.5 tsp po bid. All you have in stock is 25 mg tablets. How many tablets will you need to crush to fill the order?
    a. four tablets
    b. three tablets
    c. two tablets
    d. one tablet

30. The first four numbers of the national drug code (NDC) number represent the
    a. drug product.
    b. package size.
    c. manufacturer.
    d. dose form.

31. A patient who is allergic to penicillin may be sensitive to
    a. imipenem-cilastin.
    b. erythromycin.
    c. sulfisoxazole.
    d. levofloxacin.

32. Crash carts contain medication and equipment for
    a. patients' daily use.
    b. emergency use.
    c. physician use.
    d. sterile product preparation.

33. A pharmacy technician is filling a prescription for eye drops that reads "2 gtt od tid." How many drops will the patient use a day?
    a. 12 gtt
    b. 8 gtt
    c. 6 gtt
    d. 3 gtt

34. APAP is the abbreviation for
    a. aspirin.
    b. acetaminophen.
    c. ibuprofen.
    d. naproxen.

35. Which numbers of the NDC are specific for the drug product?
    a. middle four
    b. first four
    c. last two
    d. first two

36. The suffix that indicates a tumor is
    a. -oma.
    b. -ography.
    c. -oscopy.
    d. -olol.

37. A prime vendor agreement guarantees the wholesaler that the pharmacy will buy
    a. all brand name products direct from the manufacturer.
    b. 100% exclusively from the wholesaler.
    c. 80% to 90% exclusively from the wholesaler.
    d. all generic name products direct from the distributor.

38. The patient requests you refill her "little pink water pill." Which drug from her profile will you select?
    a. Synthroid 200 mcg
    b. hydrochlorothiazide 25 mg
    c. propranolol 10 mg
    d. allopurinol 300 mg

39. On a pharmaceutical balance, the substance to be weighed is placed on which pan?
    a. left side
    b. right side
    c. center
    d. bottom

40. Amoxicillin is available as 125 mg and 250 mg chewable tablets, 200 mg/tsp and 400 mg/tsp suspension, and 250 mg and 500 mg capsules. Which dose form and strength would you dispense for a 13-month-old child who weighs 18 lb and the dose is 25 mg/kg/day?
    a. 200 mg/tsp suspension
    b. 125 mg chewable tablet
    c. 250 mg capsule
    d. 250 mg chewable tablet

41. A patient presents a prescription for Creon-10, with directions "2 capsules ac & hs." How many capsules must be dispensed for a 3-month supply?
    a. 120 capsules
    b. 240 capsules
    c. 360 capsules
    d. 720 capsules

42. What volume of furosemide 100 mg/10 mL will you need to draw up in a syringe to equal 60 mg?
    a. 0.6 mL
    b. 6 mL
    c. 600 mL
    d. 60 mL

43. A prescription for ampicillin is ordered as follows:
    ampicillin 250 mg
    Take 1 capsule tid × 10 days
    Disp: #30
    In assessing the prescription, the pharmacy technician recognizes the
    a. duration of therapy should be 14 days.
    b. dose form is not available.
    c. prescription is acceptable as written.
    d. ampicillin should be given qid.

44. The prescription term *Rx* refers to
    a. directions for the patient.
    b. drug name and strength.
    c. symbol for *take*.
    d. directions to the pharmacist.

45. What does the term *inventory* mean?
    a. record of drugs purchased
    b. record of drugs sold
    c. list of all items available for sale
    d. value of merchandise in stock

46. Which one of the following references used by pharmacists includes not only FDA-approved indications but also unapproved uses for drugs, as well as comparative drug tables, and is updated monthly?
    a. *Drug Facts and Comparisons*
    b. *American Hospital Formulary Service* (AHFS)
    c. *Physicians' Desk Reference* (PDR)
    d. *Handbook of Injectable Drugs* (Trissel's)

47. A physician in your area regularly writes for the following compound product:

   camphor 1%
   menthol 1%
   Lubriderm lotion qsad 2 oz

   How much camphor will you need to weigh to make a pint of the lotion to have in stock?

   a. 2.4 g
   b. 4.8 g
   c. 0.48 g
   d. 0.24 g

48. Which of the following statements about investigation drugs is *true?*

   a. Investigation drugs are drugs being used in clinical trials.
   b. Investigation drugs are FDA approved for use in the general population.
   c. Investigation drugs may be ordered from the wholesaler.
   d. Investigation drugs are FDA approved for use in high-risk populations.

49. A 70 kg adult requires aminophylline IV at 0.7 mg/kg/hr. The premixed solution is 500 mg/500 mL. What is the correct rate?

   a. 0.7 mL/hr
   b. 24.5 mL/hr
   c. 49 mL/hr
   d. 490 mL/hr

50. According to the Controlled Substance Act, how many refills are allowed on a class-II prescription?

   a. five refills
   b. 6-month time limitation
   c. no refills
   d. 1-year time limitation

51. A total parenteral nutrition (TPN) order includes calcium gluconate 4.5 mEq/L. The stock vial delivers 45 mEq/100 mL. What volume will you need to prepare for a 2500 mL TPN bag?

   a. 11.25 mL
   b. 250 mL
   c. 2.5 mL
   d. 25 mL

Chapter 3

52. A reason to extemporaneously compound a product is to
    a. increase the margin of the pharmacy by making patented products.
    b. make a dose form not manufactured by a pharmaceutical company.
    c. make a supply to sell to physicians who may then sell it from their offices.
    d. make an otherwise unknown drug you think will work in humans.

53. Serum potassium levels should be checked on patients taking which drug?
    a. erythromycin
    b. sertraline
    c. valproic acid
    d. furosemide

54. The trade name for fluoxetine is
    a. Cymbalta
    b. Strattera
    c. Prozac
    d. Celexa

55. Which amendment to the Food, Drug, and Cosmetic Act of 1938 established prescription drugs and nonprescription drugs?
    a. Controlled Substance Act
    b. Durham-Humphrey Amendment
    c. Kefauver-Harris Amendment
    d. FDA Modernization Act

56. What two drugs are found in the combination product Darvocet-N 100?
    a. propoxyphene, acetaminophen
    b. propoxyphene, aspirin
    c. hydrocodone, acetaminophen
    d. acetaminophen, codeine

57. A child has to take $\frac{3}{4}$ tsp tid of a drug. How many milliliters will the child take in a day?
    a. 15 mL
    b. 34 mL
    c. 2.25 mL
    d. 11.25 mL

58. Which of the following drugs should be stored in its original container even after dispensing to the patient?
    a. Crixivan
    b. Diflucan
    c. Epitol
    d. Singulair

59. An order for 1 lb of 2% zinc oxide ointment is prepared using the pharmacy stock of 6% zinc oxide ointment and 1% zinc oxide ointment. How much of each must be mixed to obtain the desired concentration? (Assume 1 lb = 454 g.)
    a. 90.8 g of 6%, 363.2 g of 1%
    b. 363.2 g of 6%, 90.8 g of 1%
    c. 75.7 g of 6%, 378.3 g of 1%
    d. 378.3 g of 6%, 75.7 g of 1%

60. A pharmacy offers a discount to elderly patients of 10% when cash is paid for prescriptions. If the prescription regularly costs $56.75, what is the senior discount price?
    a. $56.75
    b. $5.68
    c. $51.07
    d. $62.43

61. An IV solution contains 30 g of sodium chloride in 1000 mL of solution. What is the final percentage concentration?
    a. 30%
    b. 15%
    c. 1.5%
    d. 3%

62. Which antifungal is only available in an IV dose form?
    a. fluconazole
    b. amphotericin B
    c. nystatin
    d. voriconazole

63. Which of the following drugs is an inhaled treatment for asthma?
    a. Ventolin
    b. Flonase
    c. Relenza
    d. NebuPent

64. The Controlled Substance Act requires pharmacies to purchase class-II controlled substances with
    a. DEA form II.
    b. DEA form 222.
    c. MedWatch form.
    d. FDA form 222.

65. A company that administers prescription drug benefits for covered individuals from many different insurance companies is called a
    a. comprehensive insurance company.
    b. health maintenance organization (HMO).
    c. pharmacy benefit manager (PBM).
    d. preferred provider organization (PPO).

66. A third-party payment is
    a. cash payment at the time of service.
    b. credit card payment for services.
    c. reimbursement to the patient for prescription services.
    d. reimbursement to the pharmacy for prescription services.

67. To ensure the safety of employees, hazardous drugs such as those used for chemotherapy must be mixed
    a. in a vertical airflow hood.
    b. in a horizontal airflow hood.
    c. only by the pharmacist.
    d. only by the oncology nurse.

68. Which of the following drugs is a proton pump inhibitor?
    a. cimetidine
    b. lansoprazole
    c. sucralfate
    d. metoclopramide

69. Changes in the drug formulary at a hospital must be approved by the
    a. FDA.
    b. drug utilization evaluation board.
    c. chief executive officer.
    d. P&T committee.

70. An agent that suppresses a cough is called a(n)
    a. expectorant.
    b. decongestant.
    c. antitussive.
    d. antihistamine.

71. A patient is to receive 2 L of $D_5$0.45NS with 40 mEq of KCl over 12 hours. What is the flow rate?
    a. 83 mL/hr
    b. 166.7 mL/hr
    c. 42 mL/hr
    d. 50 mL/hr

72. The USP is the official _____ of the United States.
    a. pharmacopeia
    b. material safety data
    c. formulary
    d. human resource manual

73. A filter on an IV set prevents
    a. contamination of the sterile product with viruses and toxins.
    b. air in the administration set.
    c. backflow of fluid into the IV bag.
    d. contamination of the IV solution with impurities such as glass or rubber cores.

74. The MedWatch form was developed by the FDA to report
    a. drug diversion.
    b. adverse drug reactions.
    c. violations in confidentiality.
    d. insurance fraud.

75. The generic name for Zyprexa is
    a. fluoxetine.
    b. omeprazole.
    c. alprazolam.
    d. olanzapine.

76. The name for the needlelike device inserted into veins close to the surface and used for up to 72 hours is a
    a. central venous catheter.
    b. peripheral venous catheter.
    c. midline catheter.
    d. multiple-lumen catheter.

77. A physician writes an order for a mouth ulcer formulation in a 4 fl oz bottle that contains equal parts of Maalox, Kaopectate, and Viscous Lidocaine. How much of each ingredient will you add?
    a. 30 mL
    b. 20 mL
    c. 40 mL
    d. 15 mL

78. Universal claim forms are used to
    a. process third-party claims.
    b. process a credit card purchase.
    c. return recalled drugs.
    d. purchase drugs from the wholesaler.

79. How are buccal tablets usually administered?
    a. under the tongue orally
    b. inserted vaginally
    c. between the cheek and gum orally
    d. inserted rectally

80. The measure of the number of dissolved particles in a solution and this relationship to the body's own fluid is called
    a. pH.
    b. tonicity.
    c. stability.
    d. concentration.

81. What is the vitamin administered during a Coumadin overdose?
    a. vitamin A
    b. vitamin E
    c. vitamin C
    d. vitamin K

82. How many milliliters of a 50% magnesium sulfate solution are needed to add to a TPN if magnesium sulfate 2 g/L of TPN is needed?
    a. 1 mL
    b. 2 mL
    c. 3 mL
    d. 4 mL

83. What is an advantage of using technology in the pharmacy?
    a. less need for technical help
    b. increased efficiency
    c. decreased need for pharmacist double-check
    d. increased expense

84. Which of the following items is necessary to clean up a chemotherapy leak in the hospital?
    a. emergency box
    b. latex gloves
    c. spill kit
    d. isopropyl alcohol

85. A patient with a history of peptic ulcer disease (PUD) should purchase _____ for pain.
    a. acetaminophen
    b. aspirin
    c. ibuprofen
    d. naproxen

86. What is the temperature range allowed for an item requiring refrigeration?
    a. 35° to 40° F
    b. 15° to 30° C
    c. −5° to 2° C
    d. 15° to 30° F

87. What volume of a 23% NaCl solution is necessary to make 1 L of 0.9% NS?
    a. 961 mL
    b. 3.9 mL
    c. 39 mL
    d. 25 mL

Chapter 3

88. Convert 40° F to Celsius.
    a. 8° C
    b. 4.4° C
    c. 105° C
    d. 54.2° C

89. A physical inventory of controlled substances in schedule II must be done
    a. daily.
    b. monthly.
    c. yearly.
    d. every 2 years.

90. A DEA form 222 must be filled out to purchase a supply of
    a. heroin.
    b. oxycodone.
    c. tramadol.
    d. diazepam.

91. Which drug recall is issued as a result of patient death from the drug product?
    a. class I
    b. class II
    c. class III
    d. class IV

92. What part of the computer connects the computer to a remote network via telephone lines?
    a. central processing unit
    b. operating system
    c. random access memory
    d. modem

Chapter 3

93. How should nitroglycerin (NTG) sublingual tablets be stored?
    a. in the refrigerator
    b. in a plastic weekly pill organizer
    c. in the original glass bottle with top tightly closed
    d. in an amber prescription vial with a child-resistant cap

94. How often should a patient's allergy information be updated?
    a. only at the patient's first visit
    b. once a year
    c. never
    d. at every visit with a new prescription

95. Which of the following is an example of a class-V drug?
    a. guaifenesin with codeine
    b. acetaminophen with codeine
    c. codeine sulfate
    d. chloral hydrate

96. Which of the following class-II drugs is used to treat attention-deficit hyperactive disorder (ADHD)?
    a. methylphenidate
    b. methyltestosterone
    c. methyldopa
    d. methyclothiazide

97. Milk of Magnesia is a(n)
    a. antidiarrheal.
    b. laxative.
    c. vitamin supplement.
    d. fiber supplement.

98. If the selling price of a product is AWP minus 10% plus a dispensing fee of $9.00, what will 90 Lipitor 10 mg cost if the AWP is $112.25/100 tablets?
    a. $90.90
    b. $101.02
    c. $110.00
    d. $99.72

99. How much haloperidol is in 0.75 mL of a 5 mg/mL injectable solution?
    a. 4.5 mg
    b. 3.75 mg
    c. 2.25 mg
    d. 3.5 mg

100. A pharmacy receives a prescription for the following:
    Fosamax 70 mg 1 weekly at bedtime
    Disp. #4
    Refill for 1 year
    Why should the technician question this prescription?
    a. It is a daily medication.
    b. It does not come in the strength ordered.
    c. It should be taken in the morning, and the patient should remain supine.
    d. It may only refill five times or 6 months.

101. A medication order calls for 1000 mL of a 0.2% solution. The stock solution is 1 g/mL. What amount of the stock solution will you need?
    a. 178 mL
    b. 200 mL
    c. 2 mL
    d. 0.02 mL

102. Collecting patient laboratory data, including serum creatinine and blood urea nitrogen (BUN) data, as well as a patient's height and weight, are useful in evaluating
    a. liver function.
    b. renal function.
    c. blood clotting.
    d. cardiac output.

103. What is the powder volume of a 1 g vial of drug if, by adding 3.4 mL of SWFI, your final concentration is 250 mg/mL?
    a. 3.4 mL
    b. 4 mL
    c. 0.6 mL
    d. 2.4 mL

104. A prescription is written:
    Rheumatrex 0.005 g weekly
    Disp: 1 month supply
    If the tablets are 2.5 mg each, how many will you dispense?
    a. 8 tablets
    b. 2 tablets
    c. 100 tablets
    d. 80 tablets

105. Which auxiliary label should be included on a prescription for Zyrtec?
    a. Take with food.
    b. Avoid calcium containing foods and vitamins.
    c. Take on an empty stomach.
    d. This medication may cause drowsiness.

106. Which of the following tasks is a pharmacy technician *not* allowed to do?
    a. counsel a patient about a prescription
    b. offer counseling to a patient about his or her prescription
    c. receive a written prescription from a patient
    d. update a patient's profile on the computer

107. What volume of a 0.04 mg/1 mL solution would be required to administer a 20 mcg dose?
    a. 5 mL
    b. 0.2 mL
    c. 0.5 mL
    d. 50 mL

108. A case of Ace bandages has 12 bandages costing the pharmacy $40.00. The markup is 40%. What is the selling price for each bandage?
    a. $4.67
    b. $1.34
    c. $3.34
    d. $3.47

109. The abbreviation for dextrose 5% with sodium chloride 0.9% is
    a. $D_5W0.9\%NaOH$
    b. $D_5W0.9\%NaCl$
    c. $D_5\%NS$
    d. D_5NS

110. Which of the following drugs was originally obtained from natural sources but is now synthetic?
    a. phenobarbital
    b. penicillin
    c. epinephrine
    d. vitamin B_{12}

111. Which federal agency regulates drug manufacturers that are researching a new drug entity?
    a. U.S. Drug Enforcement Administration (DEA)
    b. U.S. Food and Drug Administration (FDA)
    c. U.S. Department of Health and Human Services (USDHHS)
    d. Consumer Product Safety Commission (CPSC)

112. In which phase of clinical trials is a drug studied in a small group of healthy individuals to evaluate safety, determine a safe dose range, and identify side effects?
    a. phase I
    b. phase II
    c. phase III
    d. phase IV

Chapter 3

113. Which of the following is *not* a parenteral dose form?
    a. urethral
    b. intracardiac
    c. intrasynovial
    d. subcutaneous

114. Purchasing that is done frequently in quantities to meet demand until the next ordering time is called
    a. direct purchasing.
    b. prime vendor purchasing.
    c. JIT.
    d. ASAP.

115. Which form must be submitted to the FDA to obtain approval to market a generic product?
    a. INDA
    b. ANDA
    c. NDA
    d. patent

116. A repackaging control log contains all the following *except*
    a. internal control or lot number.
    b. drug strength and dose form.
    c. manufacturer's expiration and lot number.
    d. date of repackaging.

117. A child-resistant container is one that _____% of children under 5 years of age cannot open but _____% of adults can open.
    a. 100, 100
    b. 90, 90
    c. 80, 90
    d. 80, 80

118. Which of the following is a typical floor stock item?
    a. Maalox
    b. Lopressor
    c. Medrol
    d. Lanoxin

119. A disadvantage of the floor stock system is
    a. quick turnaround between writing the order and administration.
    b. convenience of availability.
    c. increased risk of medication errors.
    d. no risk of diversion.

120. A technician working in a drug information center might perform what type of quality assurance task?
    a. reading pharmacy literature
    b. logging information requests
    c. answering patient questions
    d. filing correspondences

121. What is the brand name for simvastatin?
    a. Zocor
    b. Zetia
    c. Xanax
    d. Mevacor

122. How many tablets are needed to fill a prescription with the Sig: 1 tablet qod, Disp: 1-month supply?
    a. 10 tablets
    b. 15 tablets
    c. 30 tablets
    d. 120 tablets

123. If a telephone caller has a question about the administration or effect of a medication, the pharmacy technician should
    a. answer the question.
    b. refer the patient to his or her physician.
    c. recommend a Web site for more information.
    d. refer the call to the pharmacist.

124. Which of the following U.S. Drug Enforcement Administration (DEA) numbers is falsified?
    a. AB1234548
    b. AB3261930
    c. AB2347627
    d. AB1928374

125. The item commonly used to sterilize instruments and equipment is a(n)
    a. filter.
    b. autoclave.
    c. biologic glove box.
    d. nuclear generator.

Chapter 3

126. The most common source of contamination when preparing sterile products is
    a. air.
    b. water.
    c. alcohol.
    d. touch.

127. Customer service is demonstrated by
    a. smiling and using eye contact when communicating.
    b. pointing to the location of items in the aisle.
    c. not putting the caller on hold when transferring the call.
    d. waiting on as many customers as possible at one time.

128. Many inpatient facilities undergo a rigorous inspection process by
_____ to maintain their accreditation.
   a. DEA
   b. FDA
   c. JCAHO
   d. DSHEA

129. What measurement is used to identify the size of an amber vial?
   a. ounces
   b. grains
   c. scruples
   d. drams

130. What is the range of gauge that needles are available?
   a. 3/8 to 6 inches
   b. 1/2 to 3 inches
   c. 13 to 30
   d. 18 to 22

131. When breaking the top of an ampule, break it
   a. away from you.
   b. toward the high-efficiency particulate air (HEPA) filter.
   c. toward you.
   d. outside the hood.

132. What is the first thing a pharmacy technician should do when a body
area is exposed to a hazardous substance?
   a. Notify the director of pharmacy.
   b. Flood the area with water and thoroughly clean with soap and
      water.
   c. Call environment service for help with cleaning.
   d. Go to the emergency department.

133. A prescription received is for 25% podophyllum, and you need to
make 30 mL. If the podophyllum costs $100/100 g, what is the cost of
the podophyllum in the compound?
   a. $25.00
   b. $30.00
   c. $7.50
   d. $75.00

134. Convert 1.5 gallons to liters.
    a. 1.92 L
    b. 3.84 L
    c. 6 L
    d. 5.78 L

135. Which of the following items is required to compound sterile products?
    a. gloves
    b. goggles
    c. short hair
    d. rubber-soled shoes

136. Which is the advantage to monitoring inventory?
    a. increase in expired products
    b. decrease in capital that is tied up
    c. increased risk of diversion
    d. need for increased storage space

137. Computerized inventory control systems automatically
    a. notify the technician about outdates.
    b. notify the technician about recalls.
    c. generate a purchase order.
    d. determine the patient's day supply.

Chapter 3

138. The signature on class-II written prescription
    a. may be stamped.
    b. may be made by the prescriber's agent.
    c. must be legible.
    d. must be handwritten.

139. Part of the on-line adjudication process includes checking
    a. for drug-drug interactions.
    b. for allergies.
    c. formulary status.
    d. storage requirements.

140. Who defines the role of the pharmacy technician?
    a. federal law
    b. state board of pharmacy
    c. department of health
    d. each individual setting

FIRST PRACTICE EXAMINATION ANSWERS

When checking your answers, review the correct answer, but understanding why the other answers are wrong may also help.

1. **Category I**
   a. Incorrect. Phenytoin (Dilantin) does not cause photosensitivity.
   b. Incorrect. Famotidine (Pepcid) does not cause photosensitivity.
   c. **Correct.** Tetracycline and drugs in the tetracycline family (e.g., doxycycline, monocycline) can cause photosensitivity.
   d. Incorrect. Levothyroxine does not cause photosensitivity.

2. **Category I**
   a. Incorrect. This number is obtained by misreading the cost as $27.95/100 capsules and then forgetting to mark up the cost.
   b. Incorrect. This is the cost of 30 capsules only without the 34% markup.
   c. **Correct.** The cost of the 30 capsules is $0.84, and the markup of 34% is $0.28; therefore add the two numbers together: $0.84 + $0.29 = $1.13.
   d. Incorrect. This number is only 34% of $27.95.

3. **Category I**
   a. **Correct.** Since 5% means 5 g is in 100 g of ointment, solve by setting up a proportion: x g/10 g = 100 g/5 g, x g = 200 g of ointment.
   b. Incorrect. Assuming that the percentage means 5 g in 1000 g, for 5%, you would make this error.
   c. Incorrect. Multiplying 10 g by 0.05 would give you this number, which is the value of 5% of 10 g.
   d. Incorrect. Multiplying 5 by 10 will produce this number, and it has no meaning to this calculation.

4. **Category I**
   a. Incorrect. The quantity would only last 1 week because the directions are to use it twice a day.
   b. **Correct.** Since *bid* means *two times a day*, the patient needs 30 mg/dose × 2 doses/day. Each capsule is 30 mg; therefore this amount is equivalent to two capsules a day: 2 capsules/day × 14 days = 28 capsules.
   c. Incorrect. This will give more than a 2-week supply and would lead to incorrect filling of the quantity that the physician prescribed.
   d. Incorrect. Multiplying 30 mg times 28 is 840 mg, which is the actual number of milligrams the patient will take in the 2-week period.

5. **Category I**
   a. Incorrect. All narcotics require child-resistant packaging unless the patient requests to use regular vial tops.
   b. Incorrect. Antibiotics should be in child-resistant containers.
   c. Incorrect. Digoxin is highly toxic if accidentally taken by children and should be in a child-resistant container unless the patient requests otherwise.
   d. **Correct.** A list of exceptions to the Poison Prevention Act includes the drug pancrelipase, as well as other agents such as sublingual nitroglycerin.

6. **Category I**
   a. **Correct.** First, solve for the cost of the 50 tablets, which is $12.43 divided by 2, which is $6.22. Then, add the dispensing fee of $6.50.

b. Incorrect. By adding the dispensing fee to the cost for 100 tablets then dividing by 2, you obtained this number, which does not allow for the full dispensing fee to be charged.

c. Incorrect. The decimal point is misplaced on the cost per tablet during the calculation process.

d. Incorrect. This is the cost of the drug without any dispensing fee.

7. Category I

a. Incorrect. Nexium is a proton pump inhibitor used for stomach and intestinal ulcers.

b. **Correct.** Cardizem is a cardiovascular agent used to treat hypertension, as well as arrhythmias.

c. Incorrect. Premarin is part of estrogen replacement therapy.

d. Incorrect. Zoloft is a serotonin reuptake inhibitor used to treat depression.

8. Category I

a. Incorrect. This is the weight of dextrose in 100 mL, as the 45% represents.

b. **Correct.** 45% means 45 g of dextrose in 100 mL of solution. Set up a proportion to determine the amount of dextrose needed for 250 mL: x g/250 mL = 45 g/100 mL, x g = 112.5 g

c. Incorrect. The percentage is mistaken as meaning 45 g of dextrose in 1000 mL.

d. Incorrect. Multiplying 250 mL by 45 does not take into consideration the meaning of percentage.

9. Category I

a. Incorrect. During the aseptic technique process, you are introducing some active drug, electrolyte, or nutrient to treat the patient.

b. **Correct.** By practicing aseptic technique you are preventing the contamination of a sterile product by a pathogen.

c. Incorrect. You may have to add water to a preparation as long as it is water for injection if it is an injectable preparation.

d. Incorrect. Sepsis is some sort of contamination by a pathogen. Asepsis is the absence of disease-causing microorganisms.

10. Category II

a. Incorrect. This would be the price for one case at the discounted price.

b. Incorrect. This would be the price for all 10 cases without the discount.

c. Incorrect. This is the total amount of money saved on the transaction.

d. **Correct.** 10 cases $\times$ \$25.00/case = \$250.00. Determine the discount (\$250.00 $\times$ 0.15 = \$37.50), and then subtract the discount from the undiscounted price (\$250.00 − \$37.50 = \$212.50).

11. Category I

a. **Correct.** Determine the amount of milligrams in the vial: x mg/20 mL = 40 mg/1 mL, x mg = 800 mg. If each dose is 80 mg, then 800 mg/vial ÷ 80 mg/dose = 10 doses/vial.

b. Incorrect. This is the calculation for the number doses in each milliliter of solution.

c. Incorrect. Arranged ratio and proportion inappropriately.

d. Incorrect. The decimal point is misplaced.

12. Category II

a. Incorrect. Methadone is a schedule-II drug.

b. Incorrect. Plain codeine is a schedule-II drug; in combination with acetaminophen, aspirin, or ibuprofen, codeine a schedule-III drug.

c. Incorrect. Opium is in deodorized tincture of opium and is a schedule-II drug.

d. **Correct.** Heroin has no accepted medical use and is a schedule-I drug.

13. **Category I**

 a. **Correct.** Ratio strength is interpreted as 1 g of epinephrine in 10,000 mL of solution; 1 g = 1000 mg. Set up a proportion: x mg/10 mL = 1000 mg/ 10,000 mL, x mg = 1 mg.
 b. Incorrect. You need to convert the quantity of epinephrine to milligrams; therefore 1000 mg is in 10,000 mL. By moving the decimal three places to the left in each number, you are left with 1 mg in 10 mL.
 c. Incorrect. The decimal is moved too far.
 d. Incorrect. If you are not going to convert the weight of epinephrine to milligrams, then you need to be more careful with decimal points.

14. **Category I**

 a. Incorrect. This mixture will only provide a 0.45% sodium chloride solution.
 b. Incorrect. This mixture will only provide a 0.3% sodium chloride solution.
 c. **Correct.** By mixing one part 0.9% NS with three parts sterile water, you will have a final concentration of 0.225% NS.
 d. Incorrect. This mixture will provide a 0.18% sodium chloride solution.

15. **Category II**

 a. Incorrect. This is the official United States compendium of drug monographs.
 b. Incorrect. This is a prescribed regimen for care of a specific disease state.
 c. Incorrect. This is the list of bioequivalent drug products established by the FDA.
 d. **Correct.** A formulary is a list of drugs selected by a committee of healthcare professionals to supply the medication needs of an institution.

16. **Category I**

 a. Incorrect. URI is not the abbreviation for urinary tract infection.
 b. **Correct.** These are the correct directions for the Sig., with the abbreviation URI meaning upper respiratory tract infection. A drug such as Zithromax would have this Sig.
 c. Incorrect. This is not specific enough; you have excluded the terms *tablet* and *by mouth*.
 d. Incorrect. The duration of therapy is missing from the directions.

17. **Category II**

 a. Incorrect. They may be next to other refrigerated products but should be in bins to contain the drug in case of a leak.
 b. **Correct.** Although having a separate refrigerator for hazardous substance is ideal, if they are to be stored with other medications in the refrigerator, then they need to be separated and stored in a bin or container that prevents a spill if an item leaks or is damaged.
 c. Incorrect. Only at the time of mixing is the drug product placed in the hood.
 d. Incorrect. A drug requiring refrigeration may not be stable at room temperature.

18. **Category II**

 a. Incorrect. The color of the final product is not a requirement.
 b. Incorrect. The inactive ingredients may vary as long as the pharmacokinetics of the final product are similar to those of the brand name product.
 c. Incorrect. To substitute a generic for a brand, it must be cheaper for the patient.
 d. **Correct.** Besides the same active ingredient, strength, and route of administration, it must be the same dose form to be considered bioequivalent.

Chapter 3

19. **Category I**

   a. Incorrect. Tiazac and verapamil are both calcium channel blockers, and a duplication-of-therapy warning should have appeared when the computer system scanned the patient's profile.
   b. **Correct.** As a technician, a duplication of therapy such as verapamil and Tiazac would produce a warning flag on the computer, and the technician should notify the pharmacist about the problem.
   c. Incorrect. The pharmacist should call the physician.
   d. Incorrect. Never discontinue a prescription without instruction from the pharmacist.

20. **Category III**

   a. Incorrect. The Health Insurance Portability and Accountability Act of 1996 (HIPAA) is the federal law guaranteeing confidentiality.
   b. Incorrect. Compliance is a patient adhering to a medication regimen.
   c. Incorrect. Medication error reporting is voluntary.
   d. **Correct.** OBRA-90 is a federal law that requires patients to be counseled by a pharmacist when picking up a new prescription.

21. **Category II**

   a. **Correct.** The P&T committee has members from various disciplines in the hospital and collaborates on policies to ensure proper medication use in the hospital.
   b. Incorrect. Human resources in conjunction with department heads establish job descriptions.
   c. Incorrect. The investigational review board will review research being done at an institution, and the prime researchers do the publishing.
   d. Incorrect. Although the P&T committee may be asked to review the medication part of a care plan, an interdisciplinary committee at the hospital will actually write the care plan.

22. **Category II**

   a. Incorrect. A pneumatic delivery system allows medications to be delivered between the pharmacy and patient floor via a tube system under pressure.
   b. Incorrect. A class-100 environment is used for sterile compounding.
   c. **Correct.** This is a machine that dispenses patient medications when requested by the nurse and verified via an interface with the pharmacy computer system.
   d. Incorrect. This is used in a class-100 environment to mix IV products with multiple additions.

23. **Category I**

   a. Incorrect. The top of the meniscus is the slightly higher edge of the concaved edge of the liquid and will give you a measurement that is too high.
   b. Incorrect. Measuring accurately to the center is impossible.
   c. **Correct.** When reading the amount of liquid in a conical graduate, the reading is taken at the bottom of the meniscus.
   d. Incorrect. This will give you a measurement that is too high.

24. **Category I**

   a. Incorrect. This represents an every-6-hour regimen.
   b. **Correct.** In hospitals, military time is routinely used to schedule medications. If the first dose is given at 0600, add 4 hours to that time for 1000 (equivalent to 10:00 A.M.) and another 4 hours to that for 1400 (equivalent to 2:00 P.M.).
   c. Incorrect. Only 3 hours after the first dose is the second dose given.
   d. Incorrect. Only 2 hours after the first does is the second dose given.

25. Category I

a. **Correct.** If 1 gr = 60 mg, then ¼ gr = 15 mg.
b. Incorrect. This amount is too high if you use the conversion 1 gr = 60 mg.
c. Incorrect. This is a ½ gr measurement.
d. Incorrect. This is a 1 gr measurement.

26. Category II

a. Incorrect. Calling patients is only necessary for a class-I recall.
b. Incorrect. Never ignore a recall.
c. **Correct.** A class-II recall does not require notifying patients who have received the product, but any stock on the shelves is to be removed and returned to the manufacturer or wholesaler.
d. Incorrect. Recalls do not get posted.

27. Category I

a. **Correct.** A DUE is a review of a medication or therapy to ensure appropriate dosing and monitoring and is usually done on medication with a high incidence of side effects and toxicity.
b. Incorrect. Although the cost may be a reason to initiate a DUE, it is not the reason in this case.
c. Incorrect. This is not a common occurrence with blood thinners.
d. Incorrect. Narcotics are addictive and have abuse potential.

28. Category III

a. Incorrect. A macrolide antibiotic, which may be difficult to dissolve, may be mixed on a nursing unit.
b. Incorrect. An aminoglycoside antibiotic, which is nephrotoxic and ototoxic, is not difficult to mix.
c. Incorrect. An azalide antibiotic is similar to macrolides.
d. **Correct.** This is classified as an antibiotic, but is an antineoplastic used to treat some cancers and should be mixed in a biologic cabinet using necessary precautions.

29. Category I

a. **Correct.** Since 1 tsp = 5 mL, then 1.5 tsp = 7.5 mL. Determine the amount of milligrams in a dose using the ratio-proportion method: x mg/7.5 mL = 1 mg/5 mL, x mg = 1.5 mg. Since the patient is to take this dose bid, 1.5 mg/dose × 2 doses/day = 3 mg/day. Use this to determine the amount needed in 30 days: 3 mg/day × 30 days = 90 mg. Given that the drug comes in multiples of 25 mg, you will need 90 mg/treatment ÷ 25 mg/tablet = 3.6 tablets, rounded to 4 tablets.
b. Incorrect. This amount will not make a 1-month supply.
c. Incorrect. This amount will not make a 1-month supply.
d. Incorrect. This amount will not make a 1-month supply.

30. Category I

a. Incorrect. The middle numbers represent the drug product.
b. Incorrect. The last two numbers represent the package size.
c. **Correct.** The first four numbers of an NDC code represent the manufacturer or distributor.
d. Incorrect. The middle numbers represent the dose form, as well as drug product.

31. Category I

a. **Correct.** Imipenem-cilastin is a monobactam that is similar to penicillin (a beta-lactam) in structure, and patients who are allergic to penicillin may be allergic to monobactams.
b. Incorrect. In many instances, a macrolide antibiotic is used when patients are allergic to penicillin.
c. Incorrect. This is a sulfonamide antibiotic.
d. Incorrect. This is a fluoroquinolone antibiotic.

32. Category II

a. Incorrect. Patients' medications are located in a separate area with easy nurse access.

b. **Correct.** A crash cart is used during a code blue or a medical emergency.
c. Incorrect. Physicians who perform special procedures may have a kit or tray in a separate storage area.
d. Incorrect. The sterile product room located in the pharmacy contains the equipment for sterile compounding.

33. Category I

a. Incorrect. This is the number of drops if both eyes are involved.
b. Incorrect. This is the number of drops if used qid.
c. **Correct.** 2 gtt $\times$ 3 times/day = 6 gtt/day
d. Incorrect. This is correct only if you use one drop three times a day.

34. Category I

a. Incorrect. The abbreviation for aspirin is ASA.
b. **Correct.** Abbreviations are used to make writing a prescription quicker. The active ingredient acetaminophen is represented by APAP.
c. Incorrect. Ibuprofen is the generic for Motrin.
d. Incorrect. Naproxen is the generic for Aleve and Naprosyn.

35. Category I

a. **Correct.** The middle four numbers of the NDC is unique to that drug product.
b. Incorrect. This represents the manufacturer.
c. Incorrect. This represents the package size.
d. Incorrect. This is not an option.

36. Category I

a. **Correct.** The suffix -*oma* is added to the route to indicate a tumor or cancer, such as melanoma.
b. Incorrect. This means the process of recording.
c. Incorrect. This means the process of viewing with the eye.
d. Incorrect. This is the nomenclature for a beta-blocker.

37. Category II

a. Incorrect. Wholesalers do not make any profit if you order direct from the manufacturer.
b. Incorrect. 100% exclusive is not possible because the wholesaler may not carry every drug a pharmacy needs.
c. **Correct.** A pharmacy signs a prime vendor contract to guarantee a certain price, and the wholesaler guarantees that a high percentage of the pharmacy's purchases will be exclusive.
d. Incorrect. Wholesalers want you to buy both generic and brand products exclusively.

38. Category I

a. Incorrect. Synthroid is for thyroid hormone replacement.
b. **Correct.** Hydrochlorothiazide is a diuretic and is a peach- or pink-colored tablet.
c. Incorrect. Propranolol is a heart medicine to control heart rate and blood pressure.
d. Incorrect. Allopurinol is used to prevent gout.

Chapter 3

39. Category I

a. **Correct.** The item to be weighed is placed on the left pan, and the weight goes on the right pan.
b. Incorrect. The weights go on the right side.
c. Incorrect. A pharmaceutical balance does not have a center pan.
d. Incorrect. A pharmaceutical balance does not have a bottom pan.

40. Category I

a. **Correct.** A suspension is a good choice for a 13-month-old child.
b. Incorrect. A chewable tablet would not be a good choice for most 13-month-old children.
c. Incorrect. A capsule is not a good dose form for a 13-month-old child.
d. Incorrect. A chewable tablet would not be a good choice for most 13-month-old children.

41. Category I

a. Incorrect. This is only a 15-day supply.
b. Incorrect. This is only a 1-month supply.
c. Incorrect. This is only a 45-day supply.
d. **Correct.** In this example, *ac* means *before meals* and *hs* means *at bedtime;* therefore the patient needs to take two capsules four times a day, or eight capsules a day. Multiply 8 by 90 days and you will dispense 720 capsules.

42. Category I

a. Incorrect. Misplacement of a decimal point one place to the left will produce this answer.
b. **Correct.** Solve this using the ratio-proportion method: x mL/60 mg = 10 mL/100 mg, x mL = 6 mL.
c. Incorrect. Setting up your proportion incorrectly will produce this answer. Remember, like units need to be on the same line.
d. Incorrect. If you say the IV solution is 1 mg/mL instead of 10 mg/mL, you will produce this answer.

43. Category I

a. Incorrect. Duration of therapy can be from 3 days to months, depending on the condition that is being treated.
b. Incorrect. Ampicillin is a capsule.
c. Incorrect. A flaw exists with this prescription, which may decrease effectiveness of the therapy.
d. **Correct.** Ampicillin is administered qid, and amoxicillin is given tid; the technician should notify the pharmacist.

44. Category I

a. Incorrect. The signa, or *Sig.,* is the directions for the patient.
b. Incorrect. The inscription is the medication and strength the physician wants dispensed.

c. **Correct.** The *Rx* symbol, commonly used in pharmacy, actually means *take.*
d. Incorrect. The subscription is the directions to the pharmacist.

45. Category III

a. Incorrect. Although you may have purchased an item once, it may not still be in stock; therefore it is not part of the inventory.
b. Incorrect. This is important to know so you can restock supply that is sold.
c. **Correct.** Inventory is the term to describe all the items available.
d. Incorrect. This is inventory value.

46. Category I

a. **Correct.** *Drug Facts and Comparisons* is the resource containing FDA-approved and nonapproved indications and comparison tables and is updated monthly, making the information always timely.
b. Incorrect. This is not updated monthly and does not have comparative tables, though it is a good reference.
c. Incorrect. This is a compilation of package inserts for brand name drug products.
d. Incorrect. This is a resource used for referencing compatibility of IV products.

47. Category I

a. Incorrect. If you calculate that 240 mL equals a pint, then you will produce this answer.
b. **Correct.** Since 1 pt = 480 mL, solve using the ratio-proportion method: x g/480 mL = 1 g/100 mL, x g = 4.8 g of camphor needed to make 1 pt.
c. Incorrect. If you misinterpret 1% as 0.01 g in 100 mL, you produce this answer.
d. Incorrect. If you misinterpret 1% as 0.1 g in 100 mL and on 240 mL in a pint, you produce this answer.

Chapter 3

48. Category I

a. **Correct.** Investigation drugs are only allowed to be used in clinical trials.
b. Incorrect. These drugs are not FDA approved for the general population.
c. Incorrect. These drugs must be ordered special so as to keep track of distribution.
d. Incorrect. These drugs are not approved for any population yet but are being studied to determine whom they are appropriate to treat.

49. Category I

a. Incorrect. The patient's weight has not been figured into the answer.
b. Incorrect. Miscalculating the concentration of the stock solution as 2 mg/mL gives this answer. Be careful when reducing fractions to the smallest denominator.
c. **Correct.** First, calculate the amount needed per hour: 0.7 mg/kg/hr × 70 kg = 49 mg/hr. Second, solve using the ratio-proportion method: x mL/49 mg = 500 mL/500 mg, x mL = 49 mL. Therefore, the rate will be 49 mL/hr.
d. Incorrect. Decimal placement problems will produce this answer.

50. Category II

a. Incorrect. Class-III through class-V drugs may be refilled five times or 6 months, whichever comes first and if ordered by the physician.
b. Incorrect. Class-III through class-V drugs may be refilled five times or 6 months, whichever comes first and if ordered by the physician.
c. **Correct.** Class-II drugs may never be refilled in a retail pharmacy.
d. Incorrect. Most states limit all other prescription products to no more than a 1-year supply of refills unless the physician orders less than a 1-year supply.

51. Category I

a. Incorrect. This is the total number of milliequivalents needed for the TPN.

Make sure to always include your units when calculating.
b. Incorrect. Not converting the 2500 mL to liters will produce this answer. Make sure all your units match.
c. Incorrect. Misplacement of a decimal point or converting the concentration to 4.5 mEq/mL will produce this answer.
d. **Correct.** Since 1 L = 1000 mL, determine the amount of calcium gluconate needed for 2500 mL by using the ratio-proportion method: x mEq/2500 mL = 4.5 mEq/1000 mL, x mEq = 11.25 mEq. Then, calculate the amount of stock solution needed for 11.25 mEq using the proportion: x mL/11.25 mEq = 100 mL/45 mEq, x mL = 25 mL.

52. Category II

a. Incorrect. Even in compounding, you cannot infringe on patent rights.
b. **Correct.** Many times, a product may be needed for a pediatric patient that only comes in tablet form, therefore compounding allows a pharmacist to make a liquid or suppository.
c. Incorrect. This constitutes manufacturing and requires a manufacturer's license, not a pharmacy license.
d. Incorrect. This constitutes an investigation drug study and must first be approved by the FDA for further study.

53. Category I

a. Incorrect. Erythromycin is an antibiotic and does not affect potassium levels.
b. Incorrect. Sertraline is an antidepressant and does not affect potassium levels.
c. Incorrect. Valproic acid has many uses but does not affect potassium levels. Patients on valproic acid who are of pregnancy age should receive folic acid though to prevent spina bifida in the newborn if they become pregnant.

Chapter 3

d. **Correct.** Furosemide is a diuretic, and all except the potassium-sparing diuretics may cause patients to lose potassium and require supplementation, requiring periodic serum potassium levels to be assessed.

54. Category I

a. Incorrect. Duloxetine is the generic for Cymbalta and is used to treat depression or neuropathic pain.
b. Incorrect. Atomoxetine is the generic for Strattera and it is used to treat ADHD.
c. **Correct.** Prozac was the first selective serotonin reuptake inhibitor (SSRI) manufactured and is the brand name for fluoxetine.
d. Incorrect. Citalopram is the generic for Celexa, which is also an SSRI.

55. Category II

a. Incorrect. This is not an amendment to the Food, Drug and Cosmetic Act; it established rules and regulations for drugs that had high abuse potential.
b. **Correct.** The Durham-Humphrey Amendment established the two classes of drugs, and it established the FDA and the need for manufacturers to submit safety data to the FDA for approval.
c. Incorrect. The Kefauver-Harris Amendment required drugs to be efficacious, as well as safe, and required manufacturers to file with the FDA before conducting clinical trials on humans.
d. Incorrect. This changed the term *legend* to *Rx only*.

56. Category I

a. **Correct.** Propoxyphene and acetaminophen are the active ingredients in Darvocet N-100.
b. Incorrect. This is the old Darvon compound formula.
c. Incorrect. This is the Vicodin or Lortab combination.
d. Incorrect. This is the Tylenol with codeine combination.

57. Category I

a. Incorrect. If the dose were 1 tsp, which is 5 mL, and was taken three times a day, you produce this answer.
b. Incorrect. If you think 1 tsp = 15 mL, you produce this answer.
c. Incorrect. This is actually the number of teaspoons a day. Be careful of the units when doing calculations.
d. **Correct.** Since 1 tsp = 5 mL, and $\frac{3}{4}$ tsp = 0.75 tsp, determine the amount of drug in a dose using the ratio-proportion method: x mL/0.75 tsp = 5 mL/1 tsp, x mL = 3.75 mL. Since the child takes the drug tid, 3.75 mL/dose $\times$ 3 doses/day = 11.25 mL/day.

58. Category I

a. **Correct.** Crixivan is sensitive to moisture, and a dessicant is in the original bottle to absorb liquid in the air that might degrade the drug.
b. Incorrect. No special packaging is required.
c. Incorrect. No special packaging is required.
d. Incorrect. No special packaging is required.

59. Category I

a. **Correct.** Alligation should be set up as follows:

6		1 part from ZnO 6%
	2	
1		4 parts from ZnO 1%
		5 parts total of ZnO 2%

x g 6%/454 g = 1 g part 6%/5 g total parts, x g = 90.8 g 6%
x g 1%/454 g = 4 g parts 1%/5 g total parts, x g = 363.2 g 1%
b. Incorrect. The quantities needed are for the wrong percentage of stock ointment.
c. Incorrect. The alligation was set up with the numbers in the wrong place.
d. Incorrect. The alligation was set up with the numbers in the wrong place, and the wrong percentage of stock ointment is selected for the quantity.

60. Category I

a. Incorrect. A discount has not been subtracted.
b. Incorrect. This is the amount of the discount.
c. **Correct.** First, calculate the discount on the regular price: $56.75 \times 0.1 = $5.68. Second, subtract the discount from the original price: $56.75 - $5.68 = $51.07.
d. Incorrect. The discount was added to the regular price.

61. Category I

a. Incorrect. Misplacement of a decimal point will produce this answer.
b. Incorrect. Dividing by 2 and misplacing the decimal point produces this answer.
c. Incorrect. Dividing the correct answer by 2 produces this answer.
d. **Correct.** Use a proportion to determine the percent of solution: x g/100 mL = 30 g/1000 mL, x g = 3 g, or 3%.

62. Category I

a. Incorrect. Fluconazole (Diflucan) is given orally and IV.
b. **Correct.** Amphotericin is only available as an IV formulation.
c. Incorrect. Nystatin is available orally, topically, and vaginally; no IV formulation exists.
d. Incorrect. Voriconazole (VFEND) is available in oral and IV formulations.

63. Category I

a. **Correct.** Ventolin is the brand name for albuterol and is a bronchodilator used to treat asthma.
b. Incorrect. Fluticasone (Flonase) is a nasal spray for allergic rhinitis. A fluticasone dose form (Flovent) is used to treat asthma.
c. Incorrect. Rimantadine (Relenza) is an inhaled treatment for influenza A and B.
d. Incorrect. Pentamidine (NebuPent) is an inhaled treatment for *Pneumocystic carinii* pneumonia.

64. Category II

a. Incorrect. This is not a real form. Roman numerals are used to classify the schedule.
b. **Correct.** DEA form 222 is a triplicate form on which to order schedule-II drugs.
c. Incorrect. MedWatch is used to report adverse events or product problems.
d. Incorrect. This is not a real form. The FDA does not control purchase and dispensing of controlled substances.

65. Category III

a. Incorrect. This is another name for an insurance company that does not have member or provider restrictions.
b. Incorrect. This is an organization that provides health insurance to members with contracted restrictions on use.
c. **Correct.** Pharmacy benefit managers administer prescription drug plans for numerous insurance companies in an attempt to provide the best service for the lowest price.
d. Incorrect. This is an insurance entity that has a defined group of physicians providing service for its members.

66. Category I

a. Incorrect. Cash at time of payment is a direct sale.
b. Incorrect. This is the same as a cash payment.
c. Incorrect. Although some insurance companies do handle reimbursements, this is not considered third-party payment.
d. **Correct.** The part the patient pays the pharmacy is the co-payment, and the amount reimbursed to the pharmacy for the balance of the payment is called the third-party payment.

67. Category III

a. **Correct.** Vertical airflow hoods protect the employee who is mixing the antineoplastic from contamination with the product; they also provide a sterile environment to compound the parenteral product.

b. Incorrect. Nonhazardous, sterile products may be compounded using effective aseptic technique in the horizontal airflow hood.

c. Incorrect. Pharmacy technicians can be adequately trained to mix chemotherapy drugs.

d. Incorrect. Although the oncology nurse is an expert on chemotherapy, the mixing of chemotherapy drugs is performed by the pharmacy staff members who have been appropriately trained in aseptic technique and handling of hazardous products.

68. Category I

a. Incorrect. Cimetidine (Tagamet) is a H_2-receptor blocker used to decrease stomach acid.

b. **Correct.** Lansoprazole, which is the generic name for Prevacid, is a proton pump inhibitor used to decrease acid production.

c. Incorrect. Sucralfate (Carafate) is a coating agent used to treat ulcers.

d. Incorrect. Metoclopramide (Reglan) is an antiemetic that promotes gastrointestinal motility.

69. Category II

a. Incorrect. The FDA approves drugs for use in humans but does not have input into individual institutional formularies.

b. Incorrect. The drug utilization evaluation board at an institution will approve investigational studies before it is started at the institution.

c. Incorrect. The chief executive officer is the president of the institution, and although he or she is concerned about the pharmacy, this person does not get involved in the day-to-day activity of the pharmacy.

d. **Correct.** The P&T committee in a hospital approves changes to the formulary to ensure that appropriate types of drugs are available to treat patients at that facility.

70. Category I

a. Incorrect. This is an agent that thins bronchial secretions.

b. Incorrect. This agent would relieve the feeling of stuffiness.

c. **Correct.** Antitussives are agents used to suppress the cough reflex either locally or centrally.

d. Incorrect. This agent is used to treat allergies, rashes, insomnia, and a wide variety of other histamine-mediated responses.

71. Category I

a. Incorrect. This is the rate if it is to run over 24 hours.

b. **Correct.** Since 2 L = 2000 mL, use the proportion: x mL/1 hr = 2000 mL/12 hr, x mL = 166.666 mL, or 166.7 mL/hr.

c. Incorrect. If the volume were only 1 L and were to run over 24 hours, you produce this answer.

d. Incorrect. This would only deliver 600 mL in the 12-hour period.

72. Category I

a. **Correct.** The USP is official pharmacopeia for the United States and contains the standards information for all approved drugs.

b. Incorrect. The MSDS is a material safety data sheet supplied by manufacturers of hazardous products and includes information on handling spills and on inappropriate use.

c. Incorrect. This is a list of available medications at an institution or prescription plan.

d. Incorrect. Each employer will establish policy and procedures relevant to that work site.

73. Category I

a. Incorrect. Filters do not remove viruses and toxins.

b. Incorrect. Air must be manually removed before starting the IV infusion.

Chapter 3

c. Incorrect. The backflow check valve prevents back flow.
d. **Correct.** The filter on an IV set is placed in line to trap contaminants such as glass or rubber (latex) cores.

74. Category III

a. Incorrect. Drug diversion is reported to the DEA.
b. **Correct.** The MedWatch form is used to report patients' adverse reactions to the drug, problems with durable medical supplies, and labeling issues.
c. Incorrect. HIPAA violations are reported to the U.S. Department of Health and Human Services or the provider.
d. Incorrect. Insurance fraud is reported directly to the insurance company or the state attorney general.

75. Category I

a. Incorrect. The brand name is Prozac.
b. Incorrect. The brand name is Prilosec.
c. Incorrect. The brand name is Xanax.
d. **Correct.** Olanzapine is the generic name of Zyprexa, which is available in tablet, zydis, or injectable dose forms.

76. Category I

a. Incorrect. This catheter is placed deeper in the body and must be placed by a physician.
b. **Correct.** A peripheral venous catheter is the most common type of IV catheter. It is inserted into a peripheral vein and for short-term administration of IV drugs and fluids.
c. Incorrect. This is a longer peripheral catheter that extends from the insertion site into a deep vein; it stays in place longer compared with other types of catheters.
d. Incorrect. This is a type of central venous catheter in which each lumen exits the catheter at a different location, which keeps incompatible drugs from mixing together.

77. Category I

a. Incorrect. This will only make 3 fl oz. Use the conversion 1 fl oz = 30 mL.
b. Incorrect. This will only make 2 fl oz.
c. **Correct.** If 1 fl oz = 30 mL, then 4 fl oz = 120 mL; 120 mL ÷ 3 ingredients = 40 mL/ingredient.
d. Incorrect. This will only make 1.5 fl oz.

78. Category I

a. **Correct.** Although most pharmacies are computerized, the computer may break down, and having some universal claim forms on which to enter insurance information is always handy while the computer wizard is working.
b. Incorrect. A special form is used for credit cards that are not processed by the cash register.
c. Incorrect. The recalled drug notice will have a form to be filled out.
d. Incorrect. A purchase order is used to order drugs from the wholesaler or manufacturer.

79. Category I

a. Incorrect. Sublingual is the term meaning under the tongue.
b. Incorrect. The vaginal dose forms include creams, suppositories, tablets, and inserts.
c. **Correct.** Buccal tablets are dissolved between the cheek and the gum.
d. Incorrect. Suppositories are the dose form used rectally.

80. Category I

a. Incorrect. pH refers to the acidity or alkalinity of a liquid.
b. **Correct.** Tonicity describes the amount of particles in a liquid. If a liquid is isotonic, it has a similar number of particles as human serum. If a liquid is hypertonic, it has more particles than human serum.
c. Incorrect. This refers to the properties a product retains over time.
d. Incorrect. This refers to the amount of product in a liquid, gas, or solid.

81. Category I

a. Incorrect. This will not help treat a Coumadin overdose.
b. Incorrect. This will not help treat a Coumadin overdose.
c. Incorrect. This will treat scurvy but does not help treat a Coumadin overdose.
d. **Correct.** The mechanism of action for Coumadin is to inhibit the vitamin K clotting factors; therefore, in an overdose, you would give vitamin K to overcome the inhibition.

82. Category I

a. Incorrect. Given that you have 50 g in 100 mL of magnesium sulfate solution, 1 mL will only provide 0.5 g.
b. Incorrect. This will only provide 1 g.
c. Incorrect. This will only provide 1.5 g.
d. **Correct.** Note that a 50% solution is 50 g/100 mL. Solve using the ratio-proportion method: x mL/2 g = 100 mL/50 g, x mL = 4 mL.

83. Category III

a. Incorrect. The pharmacy technician spends a considerable amount of time maintaining the automation technology.
b. **Correct.** Technology in pharmacy increases the efficiency of the staff in the pharmacy, which should increase the amount of time spent on clinical and direct patient care.
c. Incorrect. All work done by a pharmacy technician, even if automation is involved, should be double checked by the pharmacist.
d. Incorrect. Although expense for the automation may be considerable, it should save money in the long term.

84. Category III

a. Incorrect. An emergency box usually refers to a code blue box for cardiac or respiratory arrest.
b. Incorrect. Gloves may be necessary but not the most important.

c. **Correct.** The spill kit is a specialty kit that contains absorbent material, protective gear, and cleaning supplies for chemotherapy drug spills.
d. Incorrect. Although used to clean the hoods, this is not the best chemical for cleaning up a chemotherapy drug spill.

85. Category I

a. **Correct.** Acetaminophen does not cause gastric mucosal irritation or peptic ulcer disease.
b. Incorrect. Aspirin is contraindicated in PUD.
c. Incorrect. This is a nonsteroidal antiinflammatory drug (NSAID) that may aggravate PUD.
d. Incorrect. This is an NSAID that may aggravate PUD.

86. Category II

a. **Correct.** Refrigeration temperature needs to be maintained between 35° and 45° F and checked daily.
b. Incorrect. This is room temperature.
c. Incorrect. This is colder than refrigeration.
d. Incorrect. This is colder than refrigeration.

87. Category I

a. Incorrect. This is the amount of sterile water needed to make the NS.
b. Incorrect. A misplaced decimal point produces this answer.
c. **Correct.** Note that 1 L = 1000 mL and a 9% solution is 0.9 g/100 mL. Solve for the quantity of NaCl needed using the ratio-proportion method: x g/1000 mL = 0.9 g/100 mL, x g = 9 g. Then, solve for the amount of 23% solution: x mL/9 g = 100 mL/23 g, x mL = 39.13 mL, rounded to 39 mL.
d. Incorrect. Inverting the numbers produces this answer.

88. Category I

a. Incorrect. Inverting the fraction 5/9 to 9/5 produces this answer.

b. **Correct.** Insert the Fahrenheit temperature into the formula and solve: C = 5/9 × (F − 32): the Celsius temperature is 4.4° C.
c. Incorrect. Using the wrong formula will produce this answer.
d. Incorrect. Inverting the fraction in the wrong formula will produce this answer.

89. Category II

a. Incorrect. Although your employer may require this, federal law does not.
b. Incorrect. This is not required.
c. Incorrect. Although your employer may do this at the yearly inventory, law does not require it.
d. **Correct.** A physical inventory must be done bienially, or every 2 years.

90. Category II

a. Incorrect. Heroin may never be purchased because it is a class-I drug and has no medical use.
b. **Correct.** This is class II that must be purchased with a DEA form 222.
c. Incorrect. Tramadol is not a controlled substance.
d. Incorrect. Diazepam (Valium) is a class-IV drug and does not require a special order form.

91. Category II

a. **Correct.** Class-I drug recalls are sent when the risk of a serious event, such as death, is possible.
b. Incorrect. This does not involve death as the reason for the recall.
c. Incorrect. This does not involve death as the reason for the recall.
d. Incorrect. No such class of recall exists.

92. Category III

a. Incorrect. This is for processing data that is input before output or storage.
b. Incorrect. This is the software that allows the computer to perform certain functions.

c. Incorrect. This is the temporary, nonpermanent memory.
d. **Correct.** A modem is connected through a telephone line; the pharmacy computer is connected with a remote computer or network via the modem.

93. Category I

a. Incorrect. The moisture of the refrigerator will affect stability.
b. Incorrect. The plastic is not adequate for storage of NTG, and the drug will lose potency.
c. **Correct.** NTG is a highly volatile drug and needs to be stored in the original glass container with the cap tight to prevent evaporation of the drug or water in the air from dissolving the tablets.
d. Incorrect. The plastic is not adequate for storage of NTG, and the drug will lose potency. Also, sublingual NTG does not have to be in a child-resistant container.

94. Category I

a. Incorrect. Although this is important to assess initially, it should be updated at every visit.
b. Incorrect. This is too long, and an allergy that occurred during the year may be missed.
c. Incorrect. Allergy information is not static and needs to be updated regularly.
d. **Correct.** Every time a patient visits the pharmacy with a new prescription, the inquiry about allergies should be made.

95. Category I

a. **Correct.** Guaifenesin with codeine has the least amount of addiction and abuse potential of the controlled substances and is a class-V drug.
b. Incorrect. This is a schedule-III drug.
c. Incorrect. This is a schedule-II drug.
d. Incorrect. This is a schedule-IV drug.

96. Category I

a. **Correct.** ADHD is treated with stimulants such as methylphenidate.
b. Incorrect. This is a testosterone used to treat impotence.
c. Incorrect. This is an antihypertensive agent.
d. Incorrect. This is a diuretic.

97. Category I

a. Incorrect. Milk of Magnesia is used to induce a bowel movement, not stop one.
b. **Correct.** Magnesium has the side effect of diarrhea, and the formula Milk of Magnesia is used to treat constipation.
c. Incorrect. Although Milk of Magnesia is a source of magnesium, it is not used as a supplement.
d. Incorrect. Milk of Magnesia is not a source of fiber.

98. Category I

a. Incorrect. The dispensing fee was not added to the AWP minus 10%.
b. Incorrect. The price for 100 tablets was used, and the dispensing fee was not added on.
c. Incorrect. The price for 100 was used.
d. **Correct.** First, calculate the price per tablet: $112.25 ÷ 100 tablets = $1.12. Second, calculate the cost for 90 tablets: 90 tablets × $1.12/tablet = $100.80. Third, calculate the 10% discount: $100.80 × 0.1 = $10.08. Fourth, determine the final price: $100.80 − $10.08 discount + $9.00 dispensing fee = $99.72.

99. Category I

a. Incorrect. 0.9 mL is equal to 4.5 mg.
b. **Correct.** Use the ratio-proportion method: x mg/0.75 mL = 5 mg/1 mL, x mg = 3.75 mg.
c. Incorrect. 0.45 mL is equal to 4.5 mg.
d. Incorrect. 0.7 mL is equal to 3.5 mg.

100. Category I

a. Incorrect. This is a weekly medication.
b. Incorrect. Fosamax is available in 70 mg tablets.
c. **Correct.** Fosamax requires the patient to take the medication first thing in the morning on an empty stomach and remain supine to prevent the tablet from getting lodged in the esophagus and causing an irritation. The empty stomach ensures maximal absorption of the drug.
d. Incorrect. This may be refilled for up to 1 year if ordered by the physician.

101. Category I

a. Incorrect. Using alligation with a 1 as the stock solution concentration produces this answer. The stock solution is actually 100%.
b. Incorrect. Assuming 0.2% is 0.2 g/1 mL, you produce this answer.
c. **Correct.** Since a 0.2% solution contains 0.2 g/100 mL, use the proportion: x g/1000 mL = 0.2 g/100 mL, x g = 2 g. If the stock solution is 1 g/mL, then x mL/2 g = 1 mL/1 g, x mL = 2 mL.
d. Incorrect. A misplaced decimal point produces this answer.

102. Category I

a. Incorrect. You would monitor serum glutamic-oxaloacetic transaminase (SGOT), serum glutamic pyruvic transaminase (SGPT), and gamma glutamyl transferase (GGT) for liver function.
b. **Correct.** To evaluate a patient's kidney function, you need to know the patient's weight and serum creatinine level to calculate creatinine clearance. This is an estimate of renal function. BUN is also used to evaluate renal function by documenting accumulation of nitrogen, a waste product of metabolic activity.
c. Incorrect. You would monitor prothrombin time (PT), international normalized ratio (INR), or partial thromboplastin time (PTT) for signs of blood clotting disorders.

d. Incorrect. You would monitor blood pressure or heart rate for signs of cardiac disorders.

103. Category I

a. Incorrect. This is the volume you are adding (diluent volume).
b. Incorrect. This is the final volume once you have mixed the vial as directed.
c. **Correct.** First, calculate the volume of the final mixture: x mL/1000 mg = 1 mL/250 mg, x mL = 4 mL. Second, use the diluent volume and the final volume to calculate the powder volume: pv = fv − dv; pv = 4 mL − 3.4 mL = 0.6 mL.
d. Incorrect. This is diluent volume minus 1 mL.

104. Category I

a. **Correct.** First, convert the weekly dose to milligrams by moving the decimal place to the right three places, or 0.005 g = 5 mg. Second, determine the number of tablets per weekly dose: 5 mg/weekly dose × 1 tablet/2.5 mg = 2 tablets/weekly dose. Third, determine the total number of tablets per month: 2 tablets/weekly dose × 4 weeks/month = 8 tablets.
b. Incorrect. This is only a 1-week supply.
c. Incorrect. Misplaced decimal point one place too far to the right in converting grams to milligrams produces this answer.
d. Incorrect. Misplacing a decimal point produces this answer.

105. Category I

a. Incorrect. This may be taken without regard for food.
b. Incorrect. Calcium does not affect absorption of this drug.
c. Incorrect. This may be taken without regard for food.
d. **Correct.** Side effects of antihistamines include drowsiness. The patient should be warned of this side effect

so he or she does not try to perform tasks requiring alertness, such as driving a car.

106. Category I

a. **Correct.** The pharmacist is the individual who is allowed to counsel a patient about a drug.
b. Incorrect. Any time you give a patient a new prescription, you should offer to have the pharmacist counsel the patient about the medication.
c. Incorrect. Although each state varies on taking telephone orders, all technicians may receive a written prescription.
d. Incorrect. Anytime a patient gives you updated information, it should be added to their profile.

107. Category I

a. Incorrect. Check your conversion of micrograms to milligrams (1000 mcg = 1 mg).
b. Incorrect. The proportion was set up wrong. Remember to keep the units the same.
c. **Correct.** Since 1 mg = 1000 mcg, calculate the requested volume by using the ratio-proportion method: x mcg/0.04 mg = 1000 mcg/1 mg, x mcg = 40 mcg, or 40 mcg/1 mL. Using this volume and the ratio-proportion method: x mL/20 mcg = 1 mL/40 mcg, x mL = 0.5 mL.
d. Incorrect. Not using the right conversion will produce this answer.

108. Category I

a. **Correct.** Determine the markup cost of the case: $40.00 × 0.4 = $16.00. Add the markup to the cost of the case ($40.00 + $16.00 = $56.00), and then determine the cost of a single bandage: $56.00 ÷ 12 bandages = $4.67.
b. Incorrect. This is only the markup cost for one bandage.
c. Incorrect. This is the cost of a single bandage without the markup.
d. Incorrect. A misplaced decimal point when interpreting 40% produces this answer.

109. Category I

a. Incorrect. This is 0.9% sodium hydroxide in dextrose.
b. Incorrect. This is correct but not the commonly used abbreviation.
c. Incorrect. The percent sign is not included.
d. **Correct.** Abbreviations are used to simplify and save time; D_5NS, is used to signify a solution with 5% dextrose in 0.9% sodium chloride.

110. Category II

a. Incorrect. This drug was always synthetic.
b. Incorrect. This drug is a combination of synthetic and natural molecules.
c. **Correct.** Epinephrine is now synthetic, but it was originally from natural sources.
d. Incorrect. This drug is produced from a natural source.

111. Category II

a. Incorrect. The DEA is responsible for controlled substances only.
b. **Correct.** The FDA approves all new drug entities and studies being done on a drug.
c. Incorrect. The U.S. Department of Health and Human Service is responsible for HIPPA, among other things.
d. Incorrect. This group regulates the Poison Prevention Act.

112. Category II

a. **Correct.** Phase I is the first trial of a drug to evaluate the safety, dose range, and side effects of a chemical in healthy volunteers.
b. Incorrect. This phase is when the drug is studied in patients with the condition that it is intended to treat.
c. Incorrect. This phase is when the drug is compared with commonly used treatments.
d. Incorrect. This phase involves the post-marketing collection of data.

113. Category II

a. **Correct.** Urethral is depositing a drug into the urethra and is not a parenteral dose form.
b. Incorrect. This is an injection into the heart.
c. Incorrect. This is an injection into the joint-fluid area.
d. Incorrect. This is an injection into the area beneath the skin.

114. Category II

a. Incorrect. This is purchasing direct from the manufacturer in larger quantities at less frequent intervals.
b. Incorrect. This is a contractual situation in which a buyer guarantees purchasing a certain percentage of pharmaceuticals from a wholesaler for a special price.
c. **Correct.** JIT means *just in time*, which is the type of ordering done to keep inventory at a minimum but have sufficient stock available for the immediate needs.
d. Incorrect. ASAP is the abbreviation for *as soon as possible*.

115. Category II

a. Incorrect. This is the *investigation of new drug application* submitted for a new drug entity to start investigational studies.
b. **Correct.** This is *abbreviated new drug application* and is the form generic manufacturers submit to receive approval for a generic product once a patent has expired on the brand.
c. Incorrect. This is the *new drug application* that is submitted for drug approval.
d. Incorrect. This is filed with the patent office as soon as a manufacturer believes product is viable.

116. Category II

a. Incorrect. This is required.
b. Incorrect. This is required.
c. Incorrect. This is required.
d. **Correct.** The date the drug was repackaged is not required on the log.

117. Category II

   a. Incorrect. This is childproof.

   b. Incorrect. This is the correct percentage for adults but not for children.

   c. **Correct.** Child resistant is not childproof, and only 80% of children need not be able to open the container, but 90% of adults need to be able to open the container.

   d. Incorrect. This is the correct percentage for children but not for adults.

118. Category II

   a. **Correct.** Floor stock items in an institution tend to be items with a low risk of medication error and usage is high, such as over-the-counter products (e.g., Maalox, Tylenol).

   b. Incorrect. This is a cardiac drug that requires monitoring.

   c. Incorrect. This is a corticosteroid not used on a routine basis.

   d. Incorrect. This is a cardiac drug that requires monitoring.

119. Category II

   a. Incorrect. This is an advantage to using floor stock.

   b. Incorrect. This is an advantage to using floor stock.

   c. **Correct.** When medications are stocked on the patient unit for easy access, the risk of medication errors is increased because the checks and balance among physician order, nursing, and pharmacy is not adhered to.

   d. Incorrect. Diversion is likely to happen with floor stock.

120. Category II

   a. Incorrect. This is not a quality assurance task.

   b. **Correct.** The technician might work in drug information and help by logging in requests for information for trending at a later date.

   c. Incorrect. Only pharmacists answer patients' questions.

   d. Incorrect. Filing is not a quality-assurance task.

121. Category I

   a. **Correct.** Simvastatin is an antihyperlipidemic agent that decreases the body's production of cholesterol and is sold under the brand name Zocor.

   b. Incorrect. This is the brand name for ezetimibe, an antihyperlipidemia drug.

   c. Incorrect. This is the brand name for alprazolam, a benzodiazepine.

   d. Incorrect. This is the brand name for lovastatin, an antihyperlipidemia drug.

122. Category I

   a. Incorrect. This is only a 20 day supply.

   b. **Correct.** The abbreviation *qod* means *every other day*. Given that 30 days are in a month, then 15 tablets will be dispensed for a 1-month supply.

   c. Incorrect. This is a 2-month supply.

   d. Incorrect. This is an 8-month supply.

123. Category III

   a. Incorrect. Never answer questions requiring professional judgment.

   b. Incorrect. The pharmacist will refer the patient to a physician if the pharmacist believes doing so is necessary.

   c. Incorrect. Do not give advice about Web sites unless directed to do so by the pharmacist.

   d. **Correct.** Pharmacy technicians should refer all patient calls for information about the medication to the pharmacist.

124. Category I

   a. Incorrect. This is a legitimate DEA number.

   b. Incorrect. This is a legitimate DEA number.

   c. **Correct.** Add the first, third, and fifth digits $(2 + 4 + 6 = 12)$. Add the second, fourth, and sixth digits, and multiply by 2 $(3 + 7 + 2) = 12 \times 2 = 24)$. Add $12 + 24 = 36$. The last digit of the DEA number *should* match the last digit of the total. In this case, it does not; therefore the number is not a valid DEA number.

   d. Incorrect. This is a legitimate DEA number.

125. Category III

a. Incorrect. A filter traps particulate matter but does not sterilize.
b. **Correct.** Autoclaves sterilize using heat and pressure to kill pathogens.
c. Incorrect. This creates a class-100 environment for compounding sterile products.
d. Incorrect. This is used in a nuclear pharmacy to create isotopes.

126. Category I

a. Incorrect. Although this is a factor in contamination, it is not the most common source.
b. Incorrect. Although this is a factor in contamination, it is not the most common source.
c. Incorrect. Alcohol is used to clean the sterile field.
d. **Correct.** Human touch is the most common cause of contamination when mixing sterile products.

127. Category III

a. **Correct.** Good customer service techniques always start with a smile and making direct eye contact with the individual you are helping.
b. Incorrect. Escort the customer when possible to the location.
c. Incorrect. Telephone etiquette is important.
d. Incorrect. Although this might be considered multitasking, each customer deserves your undivided attention.

128. Category III

a. Incorrect. The DEA only inspects and monitors controlled substances.
b. Incorrect. The FDA inspects drug manufacturers.

c. **Correct.** The Joint Commission for Accreditation of Healthcare Organizations is a voluntary evaluation that institutions undergo to receive accreditation. Many insurance carriers will not reimburse if you do not have this accreditation.
d. Incorrect. This stands for Dietary Supplement Health and Education Act.

129. Category I

a. Incorrect. This is used as a measure of liquid containers.
b. Incorrect. This is not used for container size.
c. Incorrect. This is not used for container size.
d. **Correct.** Amber prescription vials are measured in terms of drams, with 6 drams the smallest and up to 60 drams.

130. Category I

a. Incorrect. This is a measure of length.
b. Incorrect. This is a measure of length.
c. **Correct.** Gauge refers to the diameter of the bore of a needle; the smaller the number is, the larger the bore will be.
d. Incorrect. These are the sizes commonly used in the pharmacy.

131. Category I

a. **Correct.** Always break an ampule away from your body and the HEPA filter but still inside the hood.
b. Incorrect. Small glass pieces can deposit in the filter.
c. Incorrect. Small glass pieces may land on you.
d. Incorrect. This will not maintain sterility.

132. Category II

a. Incorrect. Wait until you are cleaned up.
b. **Correct.** Always wash the contaminant off yourself first; then seek help and medical attention.

c. Incorrect. Clean yourself first.
d. Incorrect. Clean yourself first.

133. Category I

a. Incorrect. You would need to make 100 mL to charge this amount.
b. Incorrect. You would need to make 120 mL to charge this amount.
c. **Correct.** Since a 25% solution contains 25 g in 100 mL, calculate the number of grams of drug in 30 mL using the ratio-proportion method: x g/30 mL = 25 g/100 mL, x g = 7.5 g. Then, calculate the price using another proportion: x/7.5 g = $100/100 g, x = $7.50.
d. Incorrect. A misplace decimal point will produce this answer.

134. Category I

a. Incorrect. This is 0.5 gallon.
b. Incorrect. This is 1 gallon.
c. Incorrect. Many people think a liter is equal to 1 quart and guess this answer.
d. **Correct.** Use the conversion 1 gallon = 3850 mL = 3.85 L and the ratio-proportion method: x L/1.5 gallons = 3.85 L/1 gallon, x L = 5.775 L, rounded to 5.78 L.

135. Category II

a. **Correct.** All sterile compounding in the pharmacy should be done with gloves.
b. Incorrect. Eye protection is voluntary.
c. Incorrect. A hair cover is worn now that USP 797 is implemented.
d. Incorrect. Shoe covers are worn now that USP 797 is implemented.

136. Category II

a. Incorrect. Appropriate inventory control decreases expired products.
b. **Correct.** Inventory control is a major way to contain costs and keep health-care expense down.
c. Incorrect. Keeping stock at appropriate levels should decrease theft.
d. Incorrect. Inventory control should help limit space needed for stock.

137. Category II

a. Incorrect. It does not generate this information.
b. Incorrect. It does not generate this information
c. **Correct.** Computerized inventory subtracts when a prescription is filled, and if the inventory goes below a preset amount, an order is automatically generated to return the supply to the maximal level. The order is confirmed with a purchase order, therefore a record of merchandise that is coming in is available.
d. Incorrect. Although most computer system calculates this information, it is not part of inventory control.

138. Category II

a. Incorrect. It may never be stamped.
b. Incorrect. Only the prescriber may sign the class-II prescription.
c. Incorrect. Although this is favorable, it should appear similar to the prescriber's signature.
d. **Correct.** Only the prescriber's own hand may sign a class-II written prescription.

139. Category III

    a. Incorrect. The pharmacy's computer performs this function.

    b. Incorrect. The pharmacy's computer performs this function.

    c. **Correct.** To determine the co-pay of a prescription, the on-line adjudication is checking the drug dispensed against a formulary to determine payment.

    d. Incorrect. This information is on the product package.

140. Category III

    a. Incorrect. Federal law does not address individual roles in the pharmacy.

    b. **Correct.** Each state determines its own set of rules pertaining to pharmacy technicians.

    c. Incorrect. This is not involved in job descriptions.

    d. Incorrect. Each site must work within the laws of that state.

Chapter 3

Second Practice Examination

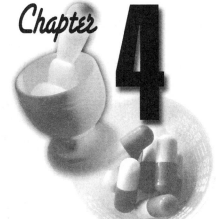

This test contains 140 multiple-choice questions. Take this test after you have reviewed the areas of technician responsibility missed in the first practice test. This test should take no more than 3 hours to complete. Read the questions and select the best answer for each question.

1. Which of the following is an example of a misbranded drug?
   a. a label that contains name and quantity of each active ingredient
   b. a label that contains adequate directions for use
   c. drugs that are dangerous to health when used in the dose or manner suggested on the label
   d. drugs that are clearly labeled with information required by the Food, Drug, and Cosmetic (FDC) Act

2. The federal law that prohibits the reimportation of a drug into the United States by anyone except the manufacturer is the
   a. Prescription Drug Marketing Act of 1987.
   b. Drug Price Competition and Patent-Term Restoration Act of 1984.
   c. Omnibus Budget Reconciliation Act of 1990.
   d. FDA Modernization Act.

3. Which statement concerning transferring prescriptions is correct?
   a. Prescription transfer between pharmacies is never allowed.
   b. Prescription transfer between pharmacies is under the control of each individual state.
   c. Prescription transfer between pharmacies may only be done by a registered pharmacist.
   d. Prescription transfer between pharmacies is under the control of each pharmacy's owner.

4. A prescription for captopril 12.5 mg #90 Sig. 1 po tid ac for CHF is presented to the pharmacy technician. Which of the following directions should be included on the label?
   a. Take 1 capsule three times a day for congestive heart failure.
   b. Take 1 tablet three times a day after meals for congestive heart failure.
   c. Take 1 tablet three times a day before meals for congestive heart failure.
   d. Take 1 tablet three times a day with meals for congestive heart failure.

5. What is the generic name for Plavix?
   a. celecoxib
   b. clopidogrel
   c. clonidine
   d. citalopram

6. Which of the following drugs is in the same therapeutic class as verapamil?
   a. Cymbalta
   b. Clozaril
   c. Cordarone
   d. Cardizem

7. Manufacturers of prescription drug samples may only distribute them to
   a. pharmacists.
   b. physicians.
   c. hospitals.
   d. pharmacies.

8. When a manufacturer of a new drug entity submits data to the U.S. Food and Drug Administration (FDA) for approval to market a new drug, the manufacturer must prove that the drug is safe and
   a. has greater potential benefit than previously marketed products.
   b. has no contraindications for use in humans.
   c. effective for the intended indication.
   d. provide data on use during pregnancy and in children.

9. Which statement regarding policy and procedure manuals is correct?
    a. Technicians should always check their employer's policy and procedure manual when unsure of safe operation of the pharmacy.
    b. State boards of pharmacy write the policy and procedure manuals that will be used in pharmacies in their state.
    c. Federal law dictates what topics will be included in a policy and procedure manual.
    d. Technicians should always do what the pharmacist tells them, even when the policy and procedure manual disagrees.

10. High levels of cholesterol in the bloodstream is a risk factor for
    a. diabetes.
    b. atherosclerosis.
    c. deep-vein thrombosis.
    d. cancer.

11. Which organ in the body is responsible for the release of insulin?
    a. pancreas
    b. adrenal glands
    c. liver
    d. thyroid

12. A patient comes in to the pharmacy and asks the technician to refill his prescription for his inhaler. He states that he is having more shortness of breath than usual and has been using his inhaler more than usual. The technician notices on his profile that he takes medication for congestive heart failure, as well as asthma. What should the technician do?
    a. Fill the prescription for the inhaler.
    b. Call the patient's physician to report an early refill of the inhaler.
    c. Suggest that the patient take more of his diuretic, and that might help his breathing.
    d. Notify the pharmacist.

Chapter 4

13. The pharmacist asks the pharmacy technician to collect liver function tests (LFTs) on all the patients in the hospital who are taking a *statin*. Which of the following laboratory test data are you collecting?
    a. serum creatinine and blood urea nitrogen (BUN)
    b. uric acid
    c. serum glutamic-oxaloacetic transaminase (SGOT) and serum glutamic pyruvic transaminase (SGTP)
    d. triglyceride

14. A patient is newly diagnosed with hypertension and asked for a product to take for a head cold. Which category of over-the-counter (OTC) agents should be avoided?
    a. antitussives
    b. decongestants
    c. antihistamines
    d. expectorants

15. The following prescription is received:
    Zithromax 200 mg tablets
    Disp: 5
    Sig. 2 stat then 1 po daily until gone
    What is wrong with the prescription?
    a. The drug should be taken for 10 days total.
    b. The drug is only available intravenously (IV).
    c. The drug is not available in this strength.
    d. The drug is only available as a capsule.

16. Which ordering technique requires the staff of a pharmacy to write down items they used so they will be reordered?
    a. minimum and maximum product levels
    b. order book
    c. inventory cards
    d. computerized inventory system

Chapter 4

17. Which of the following dose forms will deliver nitroglycerin (NTG) over a continuous 24-hour period?
    a. ointment
    b. sublingual tablets
    c. aerosol
    d. transdermal patch

18. Which of the following documents is required to practice as a pharmacist?
    a. state licensure
    b. U.S. Drug Enforcement Agency (DEA) license
    c. federal licensure
    d. high school diploma

19. Which of the following physiologic changes in older adults does not alter drug response?
    a. decreased renal function
    b. changes in gastrointestinal function
    c. hepatic insufficiency
    d. decreased hearing

20. A patient asks you if her prescription drug is available generically. Which reference would be the most useful in finding information on an AB-rated generic product for this patient?
    a. Drugs Facts and Comparisons
    b. Goodman and Gilman's Pharmacological Basis of Therapeutics
    c. FDA's Approved Drug Products with Therapeutic Equivalence Evaluations
    d. United States Pharmacopeia

21. A drug that is said to bind to a cell receptor and stimulate the same response as the body's own chemical is known as a(n)
    a. agonist.
    b. antagonist.
    c. synergist.
    d. additive.

22. Which of the following is a common symptom of *dig toxicity?*
    a. muscle aches and pains
    b. total body rash
    c. nausea
    d. angioedema

Chapter 4

23. Which of the following drugs should *not* be taken at the same time as Coumadin?
    a. heparin
    b. ibuprofen
    c. sertraline
    d. furosemide

24. Palonosetron (Aloxi) is an IV therapy to
    a. prevent nausea and vomiting.
    b. prevent organ transplant rejection.
    c. treat breast cancer.
    d. dissolve blood clots.

25. What is the name of the document with approved agents to be used in an institution or reimbursable by an insurance plan?
    a. database
    b. policy
    c. legend
    d. formulary

26. When checking in an order from the wholesaler, against which of the following documents should the order be checked?
    a. invoice
    b. want book
    c. purchase order
    d. last 24-hour usage

27. Which functions does a pharmacy technician *not* provide in relationship to OTC products?
    a. stocking shelves
    b. helping customers locate products
    c. recommending products to customers
    d. removing expired products from shelves

28. What alternative medicine might be used in place of a prescription sedative or hypnotic?
    a. chamomile
    b. ginkgo
    c. saw palmetto
    d. melatonin

29. The patient's date of birth is an important piece of information. What is *not* an appropriate use for the date of birth?
    a. third-party billing
    b. demographic information to give to marketers
    c. identifying patients with the same name
    d. evaluating the appropriateness of therapy

30. Which DEA number would be possible for a Dr. John Smith?
    a. JS1234563
    b. AS1234563
    c. BS1234567
    d. AS1234567

31. Which of the following is a near homonym or homograph, or both, of
    each other?
    a. clonidine, Klonopin
    b. clonidine, Catapres
    c. clonazepam, Klonopin
    d. clonazepam, clonidine

32. A patient buys her insulin and syringes at your pharmacy. If she uses
    52 units of insulin at bedtime, which size syringe is best for her?
    a. 0.5 mL
    b. 1 mL
    c. 3 mL
    d. 5 mL

33. A patient presents a prescription for Xanax. What is the maximum
    number of refills allowed for Xanax?
    a. none
    b. one
    c. five
    d. six

34. What special auxiliary label is required by law to be on the label of a
    controlled substance when it is dispensed to a patient?
    a. no alcoholic beverage
    b. drowsiness warning
    c. avoid sunlight warning
    d. transfer warning

Chapter 4

35. Which of the following medications requires special handling and
    preparation?
    a. fluorouracil
    b. fluoxetine
    c. fluticasone
    d. fomepizole

36. Which of the following drugs should not be touched by a pregnant woman?
    a. Proscar
    b. Prinivil
    c. Prilosec
    d. Primacor

37. The following prescription is received:
    Sulfisoxazole 500 mg
    Disp: LVI
    Sig. 2 tab po qid
    How many tablets will be dispensed?
    a. 16
    b. 56
    c. 106
    d. 506

38. If a drug vial contains 250 mg and a patient is given ¾ of the vial, how many milligrams did the patient receive?
    a. 72 mg
    b. 187.5 mg
    c. 177.5 mg
    d. 333 mg

39. The stock vial of folic acid is 5 mg/mL. How much will need to be dispensed to equal 2 mg?
    a. 0.2 mL
    b. 0.25 mL
    c. 0.4 mL
    d. 0.6 mL

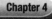
Chapter 4

40. A patient weighs 156 lb and is to receive a medication at 30 mg/kg/dose. What is the dose in milligrams?
    a. 4700 mg
    b. 2100 mg
    c. 2350 mg
    d. 2500 mg

41. Fluorouracil is dosed at 500 mg/m^2, and the patient's body surface area (BSA) is 1.56 m^2. Fluorouracil comes in a vial with 500 mg/10 mL. How many vials will you need to make the dose for this patient?
    a. one
    b. two
    c. three
    d. four

42. If a patient takes 1 tsp/dose and you dispense a 4 fl oz bottle, how many doses are available?
    a. 4
    b. 8
    c. 12
    d. 24

43. The Orange Book is used to find
    a. therapeutic equivalent generics.
    b. average wholesale price.
    c. pharmacologic information.
    d. compatibility information.

44. What is the name for the general cost of doing business?
    a. overall cost
    b. income
    c. overhead
    d. professional handling

45. Which one of the following abbreviations is considered a dangerous abbreviation by the Institute for Safe Medication Practices (ISMP) and should not be used per Joint Commission on Accreditation of Healthcare Organizations (JCAHO) accreditation standards?
    a. tid
    b. qd
    c. mg
    d. po

46. Which is *not* one of the five *rights* of filling a prescription to prevent a medication error?
    a. patient
    b. drug
    c. route
    d. container

Chapter 4

47. What is the most common reason for noncompliance?
    a. side effects
    b. forgetfulness
    c. complexity of regimen
    d. cognitive impairment

48. Which of the following is *not* a symptom of hypoglycemia?
    a. confusion
    b. sweating
    c. anorexia
    d. thirst

49. What is the most important characteristic of a parenteral preparation?
    a. sterility
    b. hypertonic
    c. alkaline
    d. nonpyrogenic

50. The instrument used to pick up weights and transfer them to and from the balance to avoid transferring moisture and oils to the weights is called a
    a. spatula.
    b. pestle.
    c. forceps.
    d. pipette.

51. The area in which a balance is used should be in
    a. the sterile product room.
    b. a low traffic area.
    c. an area of high humidity.
    d. a portable cart.

52. Which statement concerning compounding records is *true?*
    a. Compounding records are not necessary.
    b. The compounding record only requires the name of the product compounded and the preparer of the compound.
    c. The compounding record includes a record of the compounding, including ingredients, amounts of ingredients, preparer's name, and name of supervising pharmacist.
    d. A compounding record is the recipe for how to make a compounded product.

53. Typical unit dose packaging includes all the following *except*
    a. amber prescription vial.
    b. heat-sealed strip packages.
    c. blister packs.
    d. adhesive sealed bottles.

54. The laminar airflow hood should be given a thorough cleaning with isopropyl alcohol
    a. every 6 months.
    b. at the end of the day.
    c. every 30 days.
    d. at the start of the day and several times a day.

55. What is the name of the procedures used to prevent infection caused by exposure to blood or other bodily fluids?
    a. blood precautions
    b. universal precautions
    c. sterile precautions
    d. aseptic technique

56. A prescription calls for 1 pt of Bactrim Pediatric suspension to be dispensed. If the child is going to take 1 tsp a day, how many days supply is in the whole pint?
    a. 96
    b. 48
    c. 30
    d. 10

57. Prozac Liquid is available as 20 mg/5 mL. How many milliliters will you draw up if the patient is to receive 1 mg of Prozac?
    a. 5 mL
    b. 2.5 mL
    c. 1 mL
    d. 0.25 mL

58. If a patient is 5 feet, 2 inches tall, how many centimeters is the patient?
    a. 124 cm
    b. 152.4 cm
    c. 157.5 cm
    d. 62 cm

Chapter 4

59. Compounded prescriptions are priced at cost plus 30% plus a $10.00 compounding fee. If the cost of the compounded ingredients is $8.76, how much should you charge the patient?
    a. $8.76
    b. $11.39
    c. $18.76
    d. $21.39

60. When an insurer pays a monthly fee to a pharmacy to dispense all patients' prescriptions, it is called
    a. fee-for-service.
    b. capitation fee.
    c. average wholesale cost.
    d. adjudication.

61. The maximum inventory level for Cytoxan is 10 vials of 500 mg, and you use all but two vials compounding chemotherapy. Cytoxan is available from your wholesaler in packages of 10 vials of 500 mg and 10 vials of 200 mg. How many vials should you order?
    a. 8 vials of 500 mg
    b. 10 vials of 500 mg
    c. none
    d. 10 vials of 200 mg

62. What is the turnover rate if a pharmacy regularly purchases $500,000 of inventory a year and has an average inventory value of $125,000?
    a. 3
    b. 4
    c. 0.25
    d. 0.33

63. Which one of the following drugs is used in chemotherapy as a cyto-protective agent?
    a. topotecan
    b. oxaliplatin
    c. leucovorin
    d. paclitaxel

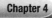

64. Which of the following toxic effects of chemotherapy causes anemia?
    a. bone marrow depression
    b. stomatitis
    c. alopecia
    d. neutropenia

65. Which diuretic is potassium sparing?
    a. hydrochlorothiazide
    b. triamterene
    c. metolazone
    d. furosemide

66. Which of the following drugs is indicated to treat Alzheimer's disease?
    a. Aciphex
    b. Accutane
    c. Accupril
    d. Aricept

67. A patient comes to the pharmacy counter and complains that the pharmacy incorrectly filled her prescription. She was suppose to get medicine to treat her high blood pressure and instead was given the same medicine her friend takes for migraine headaches. What do you tell her?
    a. "Your friend has the wrong medicine, not you, and your friend should contact her pharmacy."
    b. "Please wait while I get the pharmacist to talk to you."
    c. "Many medications have more than one use, and hers happens to be one of them."
    d. "Call your physician. He made the mistake."

68. Which of the following is an example of nonverbal communication?
    a. eye contact
    b. empathy
    c. talking softly
    d. using courtesy titles

69. When preparing capsules, which part is used to *punch* the powder?
    a. top
    b. bottom
    c. body
    d. cap

70. What size of a hard-shell capsule is the smallest?
    a. 000
    b. 0
    c. 1
    d. 5

Chapter 4

71. What size sieve will make a very fine powder?
    a. No. 8
    b. No. 20
    c. No. 60
    d. No. 80

72. What is the name of the compounded product that is a liquid in which the active ingredient is not dissolved in the vehicle?
    a. elixir
    b. suspension
    c. solution
    d. spirit

73. What is the name of the guidelines that govern extemporaneous compounding?
    a. good manufacturing practices
    b. good compounding guidelines
    c. acceptable manufacturing practices
    d. good mixing guidelines

74. Which of the following viral infections do humans get vaccinated against?
    a. human immunodeficiency virus (HIV)
    b. herpes simplex
    c. influenza
    d. cytomegalovirus

75. Which drug may only be dispensed for narcotic detoxification and maintenance at specially licensed hospitals or clinics?
    a. morphine
    b. naloxone
    c. butorphanol
    d. methadone

76. What test needs to be done weekly on a patient who is taking Clozaril?
    a. Beck's depression score
    b. serum creatinine
    c. white blood cell count
    d. red blood cell count

77. Which of the following is *not* a controlled substance to treat anxiety?
    a. buspirone
    b. meprobamate
    c. chlordiazepoxide
    d. diazepam

78. Cefepime belongs in which generation of cephalosporins?
    a. first
    b. second
    c. third
    d. fourth

79. If a patient is allergic to erythromycin and tells you that she stopped breathing once when she had it, she is also allergic to
    a. gentamicin.
    b. clarithromycin.
    c. penicillin.
    d. doxycycline.

80. What is the name of a drug also known as the United States adopted name (USAN)?
    a. brand name
    b. chemical name
    c. generic name
    d. patented name

81. When compounding sterile products, you work at least _____ inches from the edge of the hood.
    a. 6
    b. 10
    c. 12
    d. 4

82. You are instructed to make a 0.8% weight per volume (w/v) solution and you have in stock 10% w/v solution. How much stock solution do you need to make 500 mL of 0.8% solution?
    a. 460 mL
    b. 0.4 mL
    c. 40 mL
    d. 400 mL

Chapter 4

83. What is the concentration in milligrams per milliliter of a solution containing 10 mEq/mL potassium chloride? (atomic weight of potassium = 39.1; atomic weight of chloride = 35.5)
    a. 559 mg/mL
    b. 746 mg/mL
    c. 391 mg/mL
    d. 355 mg/mL

84. Which of the following drugs are measured in units?
    a. penicillin
    b. warfarin
    c. esmolol
    d. cyanocobolamine

85. Which of the following is *not* information in a package insert?
    a. indications
    b. precautions
    c. date of the most recent revision of the labeling
    d. average wholesale cost

86. Who at a typical hospital reports to the board of directors?
    a. director of pharmacy
    b. president
    c. vice president of professional services
    d. staff pharmacists

87. Which of the following duties may be done by a pharmacy technician?
    a. checking and verifying finished prescriptions
    b. receiving verbal prescriptions in person or by telephone
    c. receiving written prescriptions
    d. verifying that weighing and measuring is done properly

88. Which of the following statements about a patient's right to privacy is *true?*
    a. The medical record is the property of the facility that generates it, and the owner can sell the information whenever he or she wants.
    b. The intellectual property in the medical record is the property of the patient and can only be released with the patient's permission.
    c. The medical record is the property of the patient to remove from the pharmacy.
    d. The patient must get a subpoena to look at his or her own medical records.

89. What is the name of the branch of pharmacy that deals with the provision of radiopharmaceuticals?
    a. nuclear pharmacy
    b. clinical pharmacy
    c. community pharmacy
    d. institutional pharmacy

90. Which of the following is *not* required on a prescription?
    a. patient's name
    b. date written
    c. responsible party for payment
    d. refill information

91. What is required on a controlled substance prescription that is not on a noncontrolled substance prescription?
    a. DEA number
    b. physician's signature
    c. address of physician
    d. date written

92. For a pharmacy technician to prevent cross-contamination of solid dose forms, he or she should
    a. use aseptic technique in filling the prescription.
    b. wipe the counting tray before counting another drug.
    c. wipe the counter with isopropyl alcohol once a day.
    d. use latex gloves to handle the tablets.

93. To decrease the risk of bacterial resistance, pharmacy technicians should put which auxiliary label on antibiotic prescription vials?
    a. Federal law prohibits the use of this prescription by anyone other than the patient for whom it is written.
    b. If you are taking birth control pills, contact your pharmacist before taking this medication.
    c. Important: take all of this medication unless otherwise directed by prescriber.
    d. Take on an empty stomach.

94. To avoid precipitation, amphotericin B should be mixed in
    a. dextrose.
    b. normal saline.
    c. lactated ringers.
    d. D_5NS.

Chapter 4

95. Which of the following is a system in which a patient regulates the amount of pain reliever received by pushing a button?
    a. transdermal system
    b. intramuscular injection
    c. patient-controlled analgesia
    d. epidural injection

96. Which of the following statements is *true* concerning the DEA form 222?
   a. It is used to order controlled substances in class-III through class-V drugs.
   b. It is a duplicate form, and the first two copies are sent to the supplier.
   c. Multiple items may not be ordered per line.
   d. Anyone working in the pharmacy may sign the form.

97. Checking the temperature of the refrigerators that store medications is an example of
   a. a method to ensure proper storage of medications and avoid waste.
   b. a mechanism to control inventory.
   c. repackaging requirements.
   d. one of the five rights of filling a prescription.

98. Which of the following will cause a precipitate if added at the same time as calcium gluconate to a total parenteral nutrition?
   a. sodium chloride
   b. potassium chloride
   c. magnesium sulfate
   d. potassium phosphate

99. An example of a quality-control measure when mixing a sterile product would be
   a. turning the hood on right before starting to mix.
   b. cleaning all interior working surfaces of the hood with isopropyl alcohol.
   c. turning on the air conditioner to keep the area cool while compounding.
   d. placing all the necessary materials on a shelf behind the hood.

100. Zolpidem would most likely be ordered
   a. every morning.
   b. twice daily.
   c. four times daily.
   d. every night before bedtime.

101. Which type of insulin may be given IV?
   a. insulin lispro
   b. NPH insulin
   c. insulin glargine
   d. regular insulin

102. A physician calls and asks a technician what the dose of a drug is. How should the technician answer?
    a. Tell the physician the dose.
    b. Look up the dose and inform the physician.
    c. Ask another technician for help.
    d. Refer the question to the pharmacist.

103. What is the proper way to write *five milligrams* to prevent a medication error?
    a. 5.0 mg
    b. 5 mg
    c. 0.5 mg
    d. 0.005 g

104. A prescription for Serevent Diskus is received with the Sig. 1 bid. What is the appropriate direction to type on the label?
    a. Take 1 dose twice a day.
    b. Inhale 1 dose two times a day.
    c. Inhale 1 puff by mouth two times a day.
    d. Take 1 capsule twice a day.

105. The name of a machine used to add micronutrients to an IV solution is
    a. Pyxis
    b. a pneumatic tube
    c. Soluset
    d. Micromix admixture compounder

106. Communication requires verbal skills, as well as
    a. professional judgment.
    b. listening to speakers.
    c. direct eye contact.
    d. multilingual abilities.

Chapter 4

107. Which of the following pregnancy risk levels means the drug is a definite risk?
    a. A
    b. C
    c. D
    d. X

108. Which of the following purchasing methods enable a pharmacy to use a single source to purchase numerous products from numerous manufacturers?
   a. direct purchasing
   b. wholesaler purchasing
   c. just in time purchasing
   d. independent purchasing

109. What federal act established the National Drug Code (NDC)?
   a. Durham-Humphrey Amendment
   b. Drug Listing Act
   c. Prescription Drug Marketing Act
   d. Health Insurance Portability and Accountability Act

110. The rebound phenomenon called rhinitis medicamentosa occurs with prolonged use of
   a. antihistamines.
   b. antitussives.
   c. antihypertensives.
   d. decongestants.

111. A patient taking the antibiotic metronidazole should be told to avoid
   a. dairy products.
   b. driving.
   c. sunlight.
   d. alcohol.

112. The name for an infection acquired while in the hospital is
   a. nosocomial.
   b. empirical.
   c. aerobic.
   d. superinfection.

113. If the record keeping for controlled substances is not up to date, which agency is charged with enforcement?
   a. FDA
   b. Consumer Product Safety Commission
   c. DEA
   d. U.S. Department of Health and Human Services

114. Which medication is used to treat gout?
   a. acetaminophen
   b. acetazolamide
   c. acarbose
   d. allopurinol

115. The term used to describe having more receipts than expenses is
    a. turnover.
    b. profit.
    c. markup.
    d. dispensing fee.

116. Which of the following is a reason for a manufacturer to recall a drug?
    a. contamination
    b. low profits
    c. label change
    d. change in advertising

117. When receiving an order from the wholesaler, all of the following should be checked *except*
    a. name of product.
    b. product strength.
    c. quantity.
    d. cost.

118. When stocking pharmaceuticals received, always place shortest expiration dated products
    a. behind other stock.
    b. on the counter.
    c. in front of the other stock.
    d. next to the other stock.

119. A medication order says to give the patient 30 mL of Mylanta II. How many fluid ounces is this?
    a. 0.5 fl oz
    b. 1 fl oz
    c. 2 fl oz
    d. 4 fl oz

120. Which of the following units of weight is used in the apothecary system?
    a. milliliter
    b. milligram
    c. tablespoon
    d. grain

Chapter 4

121. If a product on formulary is not available from the manufacturer in unit-dose packaging, the technician should
    a. recommend it be taken off the formulary.
    b. order bulk and repackage in unit-dose packaging.
    c. order bulk and send bulk package to the floor for patient use.
    d. interchange with a therapeutic equivalent drug available unit dosed.

122. Which of the following medications must be refrigerated after dispensing?
    a. cephalexin pediatric suspension
    b. sulfamethoxazole and trimethoprim pediatric suspension
    c. Dilantin pediatric suspension
    d. Prozac liquid

123. Information on how to handle hazardous substance at your facility might be found in a
    a. compounding logbook.
    b. repackaging logbook.
    c. policy and procedure manual.
    d. human resource manual.

124. What is the name of the rigorous inspection process with JCAHO that institutions voluntarily submit?
    a. registration
    b. licensure
    c. certification
    d. accreditation

125. A patient is being started on a heparin drip at 10 units/kg/hr and weighs 210 lb. If the stock solution is 25,000 units/500 mL, what rate will the IV solution run?
    a. 42 mL/hr
    b. 19.1 mL/hr
    c. 38 mL/hr
    d. 1.9 mL/hr

126. When updating a patient profile, which of the following would a technician *not* ask a patient?
    a. changes in insurance coverage
    b. OTC medications the patient takes regularly
    c. drug allergies
    d. addiction history

127. In the following prescription, how many tablets should be dispensed?

Prednisone 10 mg
1 tab qid × 4 days
1 tab tid × 4 days
1 tab bid × 2 days
1 tab daily × 2 days
½ tab daily × 2 days

a. 14
b. 42
c. 35
d. 40

128. A prescription for Patanol reads *ou*. What do you type on the label?

a. both ears
b. both eyes
c. right eye
d. right ear

129. A female patient comes in with a prescription that could be either Proscar or ProSom Sig. 1 po qhs. How do you know it is ProSom?

a. Proscar is for benign prostate hyperplasia, and only men take it.
b. ProSom is an estrogen, and only women take it.
c. ProSom is for sleep and is taken at bedtime.
d. Proscar is taken qid.

130. Which of the following is exempt from the Poison Prevention Act?

a. hormone replacement therapy
b. oral contraceptives in the manufacturer's dispensing package
c. isosorbide mononitrate
d. potassium chloride tablets

131. Xalatan should be stored before dispensing

a. at room temperature.
b. in the freezer.
c. in the controlled substance cabinet.
d. in the refrigerator.

132. Which of the following terms means the act of reducing a substance to a small, fine particle?

a. blending
b. comminution
c. trituration
d. spatulation

133. For what purpose is a master formula sheet used?
    a. purchasing drugs
    b. pricing prescriptions
    c. compounding medications
    d. filling medication orders

134. All the following are bases used to make suppositories *except*
    a. lactose.
    b. cocoa butter.
    c. hydrogenated vegetable oils.
    d. glycerinated gelatin.

135. A therapeutic use for a radiopharmaceutical is
    a. imaging regional function of the thyroid gland.
    b. treating hyperthyroidism.
    c. treating hypothyroidism.
    d. imaging broken bones.

136. Who has regulatory oversight of the practice of pharmacy?
    a. National Association of Boards of Pharmacy (NABP)
    b. FDA
    c. DEA
    d. state board of pharmacy

137. The Dietary Supplement Health and Education Act established
    a. FDA oversight of the nutritional supplement market.
    b. that the FDA did not have over site over the nutritional supplement market.
    c. that manufacturers may make health claims to sell their products.
    d. that the proof of benefit lies with the manufacturer.

Chapter 4

138. Which of the following is the brand name for capecitabine?
    a. Xanax
    b. Zantac
    c. Xeloda
    d. Zoladex

139. A patient only wishes to purchase $10.00 worth of his prescription. If 100 tablets cost $29.79, how many tablets will you sell him?
    a. 33 tablets
    b. 30 tablets
    c. 35 tablets
    d. none

140. Which word means to inhibit growth of bacteria?
a. bactericidal
b. disinfectant
c. aseptic
d. bacteriostatic

SECOND PRACTICE EXAMINATION ANSWERS

When checking your answers, review the correct answer, but understanding why the other answers are wrong may also help.

1. **Category I**
   a. Incorrect. The label must contain the name and quantity of the active ingredients.
   b. Incorrect. The law requires adequate directions for use.
   c. **Correct.** Misbranded includes labeling that may harm a patient if the medication is taken in the manner directed on the label.
   d. Incorrect. The FDCA is the Act that first required labeling and defined misbranded drugs.

2. **Category I**
   a. **Correct.** This law is under scrutiny in recent years because senior citizens trying to save money on prescriptions are traveling to Canada and Mexico to purchase prescription drugs.
   b. Incorrect. This Act helps streamline the process for generic approval and extended patent licenses.
   c. Incorrect. This Act requires states that participate in Medicaid to establish standards of practice for pharmacists, including counseling patients and reviewing drug use.
   d. Incorrect. This Act updates the labeling currently on prescription medications to *Rx only*.

3. **Category I**
   a. Incorrect. Although this may be the law in some states, it is not in others.
   b. **Correct.** Each state board of pharmacy determines if transferring prescriptions between pharmacies is allowed and the manner in which this process will take place.
   c. Incorrect. Although this may be the law in some states, others allow pharmacy technicians to transfer prescriptions.

   d. Incorrect. An owner may choose not to participate in transfer of prescription, but the state rules and regulations establish the legality of this activity.

4. **Category I**
   a. Incorrect. Captopril is a tablet, and the abbreviation *ac* was not included.
   b. Incorrect. The *ac* means *before meals*, not after meals. Food decreases the absorption of the drug.
   c. **Correct.** The abbreviations *po, ac, tid,* and *CHF* stand for *by mouth, before meals, three times a day,* and *congestive heart failure,* respectively.
   d. Incorrect. The *ac* means *before meals,* not with meals.

5. **Category I**
   a. Incorrect. Celebrex is the brand name of celecoxib.
   b. **Correct.** Plavix is the brand name for clopidogrel, an antiplatelet drug.
   c. Incorrect. Catapres is the brand name of clonidine.
   d. Incorrect. Celexa is the brand name of citalopram.

6. **Category I**
   a. Incorrect. Cymbalta is an antidepressant, not a calcium channel blocker.
   b. Incorrect. Clozaril is an antipsychotic, not a calcium channel blocker.
   c. Incorrect. Cordarone is an antiarrhythmic, not a calcium channel blocker.
   d. **Correct.** Cardizem and verapamil are both calcium channel blockers.

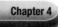
Chapter 4

7. **Category II**

   a. Incorrect. Only individuals with a license to prescribe can sign for prescription drug samples.
   b. **Correct.** Only prescribers of prescription drugs may receive samples.
   c. Incorrect. Must be an individual prescriber.
   d. Incorrect. Must be an individual prescriber.

8. **Category II**

   a. Incorrect. The potential benefit only helps the FDA decide how quickly it should review the application.
   b. Incorrect. Potential benefit must always be weighed against risk, and not all drugs are safe for all patients.
   c. **Correct.** Effectiveness for the indication for which the manufacturer intends to market the drug must be proven.
   d. Incorrect. Although this data would be useful, it is seldom done because of the high risk of studying drugs in these populations.

9. **Category III**

   a. **Correct.** As an employee, anytime you are not sure of the appropriate procedure to follow, the policy and procedure manual should be checked for directions.
   b. Incorrect. Relevant state and federal laws are taken into consideration when writing policy and procedures, but each employer writes his or her own manual.
   c. Incorrect. No federal law exists dictating anything about a policy and procedure manual.
   d. Incorrect. Technicians should be aware of the policy and procedure manual and follow the guidelines established in it.

10. **Category I**

   a. Incorrect. Although high cholesterol may be secondary to diabetes, it does not cause diabetes.

   b. **Correct.** Artherosclerosis is the accumulation of fats in the arteries and clogging the vessels and limiting blood flow.
   c. Incorrect. Blood pooling from inactivity causes most cases of deep-vein thrombosis.
   d. Incorrect. Cholesterol has not been linked to cancer, though a diet high in fat has been.

11. **Category I**

   a. **Correct.** Insulin is made, stored, and released from the pancreas.
   b. Incorrect. The adrenal glands produce catecholamines and steroid hormones.
   c. Incorrect. The liver is responsible for metabolism.
   d. Incorrect. The thyroid hormone is produced by the thyroid.

12. **Category I**

   a. Incorrect. The patient may have symptoms of worsening congestive heart failure, not the asthma. The patient needs to talk to his physician.
   b. Incorrect. Although this would notify the physician that something of importance is going on, the pharmacist should handle this situation.
   c. Incorrect. Although this may be what the physician may order, it is not up to the technician to use professional judgment and prescribe.
   d. **Correct.** The pharmacist should be notified and may be able to direct the patient to a more appropriate approach to dealing with the shortness of breath.

13. **Category I**

   a. Incorrect. This is a measure of renal function.
   b. Incorrect. Uric acid is evaluated in gout.
   c. **Correct.** SGOT and SGTP are liver enzymes and are used to access the damage to the liver.

Chapter 4

d. Incorrect. Triglycerides are measured as part of a lipid panel.

14. Category I

a. Incorrect. Cough suppressants do not affect blood pressure.
b. **Correct.** Decongestants can increase heart rate and blood pressure and should be avoided by patients with hypertension or heart disease.
c. Incorrect. Antihistamines do not affect blood pressure.
d. Incorrect. Expectorants do not affect blood pressure.

15. Category I

a. Incorrect. The Zithromax Z-PAK is a 5-day therapy.
b. Incorrect. The drug is available in IV and oral dose forms.
c. **Correct.** The drug is not available in this strength but in 250 mg tablets.
d. Incorrect. It is a tablet dose form.

16. Category II

a. Incorrect. This system's predetermined levels decide if the item will be reordered.
b. **Correct.** An order book is a system used to reorder drugs used during the day and requires anyone who fills a prescription or sells an item to write down the information.
c. Incorrect. Inventory cards establish an ongoing history of drug use and purchase.
d. Incorrect. The computer is programmed to order stock when a prescription is filled and when the predetermined minimum is reached.

17. Category II

a. Incorrect. NTG ointment last approximately 4 to 6 hours.
b. Incorrect. NTG sublingual tablets have immediate affect and a short duration of action.
c. Incorrect. NTG aerosol is also for immediate effect and has a short duration of action.

d. **Correct.** The NTG patch is designed to deliver the drug continuously for 24 hours while it is worn. Many physicians will have patients remove the patch at bedtime to give them a drug-free interval, which helps decrease the development of tolerance to the drug.

18. Category III

a. **Correct.** A pharmacist must graduate from an accredited college of pharmacy, complete an internship, and pass a standardized examination before receiving licensure to practice as a pharmacist in a state. Each state's rule may vary slightly in this procedure.
b. Incorrect. To prescribe and dispense controlled substances, a DEA license is required.
c. Incorrect. No federal license for pharmacists exists.
d. Incorrect. Although necessary for college, this is not on the list of state licensure requirements.

19. Category I

a. Incorrect. Altered renal function can decrease drug elimination.
b. Incorrect. Changes in gastrointestinal function can affect absorption of drugs.
c. Incorrect. Liver metabolism of drugs may be altered in hepatic disease.
d. **Correct.** Although communicating with patients may take time, drug response is not altered.

20. Category I

a. Incorrect. Although this contains a wealth of information, it does not contain ratings for generics.
b. Incorrect. This is useful to the pharmacist in answering clinical questions about how drugs work.
c. **Correct.** This is the long name for the FDA's *Orange Book,* which is an electronic reference to evaluate the bioequivalence of generic products.

d. Incorrect. This is the national standard for drug substances and dose forms.

21. Category I

a. **Correct.** A drug that is an agonist will simulate a receptor similar to the body's own stimulus.
b. Incorrect. These block the action of the body's receptors.
c. Incorrect. This is a term meaning that the additive effect of two drugs together is greater than either drug alone.
d. Incorrect. This means that a drug has additional effect if added to therapy.

22. Category I

a. Incorrect. This is a rare reaction that can occur to patients on statins.
b. Incorrect. Rashes are usually signs of an allergic reaction.
c. **Correct.** Nausea, as well as visual changes, is one of the earliest signs of digoxin toxicity.
d. Incorrect. This is a rare allergic reaction to angiotensin-converting enzyme (ACE) inhibitors.

23. Category I

a. Incorrect. Actually, patients may take heparin for a few days with Coumadin while the dose is being adjusted.
b. **Correct.** Ibuprofen is a nonsteroidal antiinflammatory drug and may cause some antiplatelet activity, as well as gastric or duodenal ulcers that are highly prone to bleeding.
c. Incorrect. No drug interaction is identified.
d. Incorrect. No drug interaction is identified.

24. Category I

a. **Correct.** This is one of the agents used before chemotherapy to prevent nausea and vomiting, which the antineoplastic may cause.
b. Incorrect. This use is not indicated.

c. Incorrect. This drug is given before starting therapy to treat cancer.
d. Incorrect. This drug is not indicated as a fibrinolytic.

25. Category II

a. Incorrect. A database is a computer file of information.
b. Incorrect. A policy is a guideline for a given procedure.
c. Incorrect. A legend is the *Rx only* on the prescription drug bottle.
d. **Correct.** A formulary is an approved list of drug for an institution or prescription insurance plan.

26. Category II

a. Incorrect. This document helps identify if the pharmacy was charged appropriately for items in the order but may differ from items actually ordered if they are out of stock.
b. Incorrect. This is not an effective document.
c. **Correct.** By checking the order that came in against the purchase order, you will make sure all the items you ordered are received, preventing a shortage later on.
d. Incorrect. The volume of pharmaceuticals used in a pharmacy daily does not make this an option.

27. Category III

a. Incorrect. Technicians do this job.
b. Incorrect. Technicians help customers locate products.
c. **Correct.** Selecting an item for a particular medical problem should be done by the pharmacist.
d. Incorrect. Technicians do this job.

28. Category I

a. Incorrect. This may be effective as an antiflatulent.
b. Incorrect. This may be an effective circulatory stimulant.
c. Incorrect. This may be useful for prostate health.

d. **Correct.** Melatonin is a dietary supplement that has sedating qualities similar to eating a large meal.

29. Category I

a. Incorrect. All third-party billing requires a date of birth.
b. **Correct.** The Health Insurance Portability and Accountability Act of 1996 (HIPAA) prevents the use of any private information collected by a pharmacy to be used for marketing reasons unless the patient is notified of such use.
c. Incorrect. Many times, this is the easiest way to identify different individuals.
d. Incorrect. Pharmacist can sometimes tell by the person's age that a drug is not indicated.

30. Category I

a. Incorrect. DEA numbers start with A or B.
b. **Correct.** Given that Mr. Smith is a medical physician, the DEA number starts with an A or a B; then, by putting the numbers in the validation formula, this is a valid DEA number.
c. Incorrect. These two names are equivalent; one is the brand name, and the other is the generic name.
d. Incorrect. These two names are equivalent; one is the brand name, and the other is the generic name.

31. Category I

a. **Correct.** Sound-alike–look-alike drugs (SALADs) are responsible for medication errors resulting from the similarity in the names.
b. Incorrect. These two names are not commonly confused.
c. Incorrect. These two names are not commonly confused.
d. Incorrect. These two names are not commonly confused.

32. Category I

a. Incorrect. Given that insulin is usually 100 units/mL, this syringe would require her to administer two injections.
b. **Correct.** Insulin is 100 units/mL; therefore she will need to inject 0.52 mL to get the dose, and she will need a 1 mL syringe with appropriate markings.
c. Incorrect. Insulin is never administered with a syringe this big.
d. Incorrect. Insulin is never administered with a syringe this big.

33. Category I

a. Incorrect. The Controlled Substances Act (CSA) allows a maximum of five refills or 6 months, whichever comes first. Only class-II drugs cannot be refilled.
b. Incorrect. The CSA allows a maximum of five refills or 6 months, whichever comes first.
c. **Correct.** The CSA allows a maximum of five refills or 6 months, whichever comes first.
d. Incorrect. The CSA allows a maximum of five refills or 6 months, whichever comes first.

34. Category II

a. Incorrect. This warning is not federally required but is an important counseling point for the patient.
b. Incorrect. This warning is not federally required but is an important counseling point for the patient.
c. Incorrect. This is not a necessary warning on most controlled substances.
d. **Correct.** The transfer warning advises the patient that this prescription is only for the individual whose name is on the bottle.

35. Category II

a. **Correct.** Fluorouracil is an antineoplastic and needs to be handled as a hazardous substance, with strict adherence to handling and preparation precautions.

Chapter 4

b. Incorrect. This is the generic name for Prozac, a selective serotonin reuptake inhibitor.

c. Incorrect. This is the generic name for Flovent and Flonase, a corticosteroid.

d. Incorrect. This is the generic name for Antizol.

36. Category II

a. **Correct.** Proscar (finasteride) is an antitestosterone drug, which, if taken by a pregnant woman, may harm a male fetus.

b. Incorrect. External contact does not affect the fetus.

c. Incorrect. External contact does not affect the fetus.

d. Incorrect. External contact does not affect the fetus.

37. Category I

a. Incorrect. This would be XVI in roman numerals.

b. **Correct.** Since L = 50, V = 5, and I = 1, LVI tablets = 50 + 5 + 1 = 56 tablets.

c. Incorrect. This would be CVI in roman numerals.

d. Incorrect. This would be DVI in roman numerals.

38. Category I

a. Incorrect. This is $\frac{1}{4}$ of the vial.

b. **Correct.** Since $\frac{3}{4}$ vial = 0.75 vial, solve using the ratio-proportion method: x mg/0.75 vial = 250 mg/1 vial, x mg = 187.5 mg.

c. Incorrect. A mathematical error produces this answer.

d. Incorrect. This is more than the original vial contains.

39. Category I

a. Incorrect. This would only be 1 mg of folic acid.

b. Incorrect. This would be 1.25 mg of folic acid.

c. **Correct.** Solve using the ratio-proportion method: x mL/2 mg = 1 mL/5 mg, x mL = 0.4 mL.

d. Incorrect. This would be 3 mg of folic acid.

40. Category I

a. Incorrect. Failing to convert the weight to kilograms produces this answer.

b. **Correct.** Convert the patient's weight to kilograms: 156 lb $\times$ 1 kg/2.2 lb = 70.9 kg. Calculate the dose: 70.9 kg $\times$ 30 mg/kg/dose = 2127 mg/dose.

c. Incorrect. Using the incorrect conversion of pounds to kilogram produces this answer.

d. Incorrect. This would be closer to a 35 mg/kg dose.

41. Category I

a. Incorrect. The patient will need 780 mg; therefore one vial does not contain enough drug.

b. **Correct.** Multiply the dose by the BSA (500 mg/m^2 $\times$ 1.56 m^2 = 780 mg). Given that only 500 mg is in a vial, you will need two vials.

c. Incorrect. These are too many vials.

d. Incorrect. These are too many vials.

42. Category I

a. Incorrect. Using the conversion, 1 tsp = 5 mL and 1 fl oz = 30 mL, this answer is not even close.

b. Incorrect. Using the wrong conversion for teaspoons produces this answer.

c. Incorrect. Using the wrong conversion for ounces produces this answer.

d. **Correct.** Since 1 tsp = 5 mL and 1 fl oz = 30 mL, first determine the amount of milliliters in the bottle using the ratio-proportion method: x mL/4 fl oz = 30 mL/1 fl oz, x mL = 120 mL. Second, determine the number of doses in 120 mL: x doses/120 mL = 1 dose/5 mL, x doses = 24 doses.

43. Category II

a. **Correct.** This is the electronic book published by the FDA to list approved generic equivalents.

Chapter 4

b. Incorrect. The *Red Book* would help find this information.

c. Incorrect. A resource such as *Goodman and Gilman's Pharmacological Basis of Therapeutics* would contain this information.

d. Incorrect. Resources such as *Trissel's Stability of Compounded Formulations* or *King's Guide for Parenteral Products* would give this information.

44. Category II

a. Incorrect. Overall cost is the cost of the product plus the cost to dispense the product.

b. Incorrect. Income is the overhead plus profit received by the pharmacy.

c. **Correct.** Overhead includes items (e.g., payroll, utilities, maintenance) that are required to function as a business.

d. Incorrect. Professional handling is the processing and recording of the prescription, as well as patient consultation.

45. Category III

a. Incorrect. *tid* is not considered a dangerous abbreviation.

b. **Correct.** *qd* is on the unacceptable list of abbreviations because it may be confused with *qid* when written in haste.

c. Incorrect. *mg* is not considered a dangerous abbreviation.

d. Incorrect. *po* is not considered a dangerous abbreviation.

46. Category I

a. Incorrect. This is one of the five rights.

b. Incorrect. This is one of the five rights.

c. Incorrect. This is one of the five rights.

d. **Correct.** Although it is important to put the drug in the right container, it is not one of the five rights that must be followed to prevent medication errors.

47. Category I

a. **Correct.** Patients will not be compliant with a drug that is causing side effects.

b. Incorrect. Although this is a component, it is not the most common reason.

c. Incorrect. Although this is a component, it is not the most common reason.

d. Incorrect. Although this is a component, it is not the most common reason.

48. Category I

a. Incorrect. This is a symptom of hypoglycemia.

b. Incorrect. This is a symptom of hypoglycemia.

c. **Correct.** Anorexia is not a sign of hypoglycemia but is a sign of digoxin and theophylline toxicity.

d. Incorrect. This is a symptom of hypoglycemia.

49. Category I

a. **Correct.** A parenteral product must always be sterile because it is being injected directly into the body.

b. Incorrect. Isotonic is the preferred tonicity of a parenteral product.

c. Incorrect. A neutral pH is the preferred pH of a parenteral product.

d. Incorrect. Nonpyrogenic is important for IV solutions but is not as important compared with sterility.

50. Category I

a. Incorrect. Spatulas are used to transfer solid materials to the weighing pans.

b. Incorrect. The pestle is used to grind or mix ingredients in a mortar.

c. **Correct.** Forceps or tweezers is the name for the tool to transfer weights.

d. Incorrect. A pipette is long, thin, calibrated glass tube for measuring liquid volumes less than 1.5 mL.

Chapter 4

51. **Category I**

    a. Incorrect. Only products for mixing sterile products should be in the sterile product room.
    b. **Correct.** Nonsterile compounding should be done in an area of low traffic to avoid air turbulence that may alter the balance's ability to weigh accurately.
    c. Incorrect. The balance should be in an area of low humidity to prevent water damage.
    d. Incorrect. The balance should be used and stored on a secure, level counter.

52. **Category II**

    a. Incorrect. Some sort of record keeping is required for compounding.
    b. Incorrect. The ingredients and supervising pharmacist's name are also required.
    c. **Correct.** A compounding record should provide all the information someone would need to recreate the compounded product plus information on the products used in case of a recall.
    d. Incorrect. Although it may contain this information, it must also have the information listed in the correct answer as well.

53. **Category II**

    a. **Correct.** Amber prescription bottles are considered bulk and not unit dose.
    b. Incorrect. This is a type of unit-dose packaging used for solid dose forms.
    c. Incorrect. This is a type of unit-dose packaging used for solid dose forms.
    d. Incorrect. This is a type of unit-dose packaging used for liquids.

54. **Category III**

    a. Incorrect. The hood should be cleaned at least daily; an outside firm should inspect the hood every 6 months to make sure it is working properly.

    b. Incorrect. This does not help decrease contamination risk during the workday.
    c. Incorrect. This is a good answer.
    d. **Correct.** USP 797 requires the hood to be wiped with isopropyl alcohol at the beginning and numerous times during the day to prevent contamination of sterile products.

55. **Category I**

    a. Incorrect. Blood is not the only fluid that contains pathogens.
    b. **Correct.** Universal precautions should be used anytime a healthcare professional might be exposed to contaminated bodily fluids, and all patient fluids are considered contaminated.
    c. Incorrect. Sterility is not the only way to prevent transfer of pathogens from one individual to another.
    d. Incorrect. This is the procedure used to make sterile products for patient use.

56. **Category I**

    a. **Correct.** Since 1 pt = 480 mL and 1 tsp = 5 mL, determine the number of doses in a pint by using the ratio-proportion method: x doses/480 mL = 1 dose/5 mL, x doses = 96 doses. Since the patient takes 1 dose/day, 1 pt will last 96 days.
    b. Incorrect. This would only be 1 cup of Bactrim, or 240 mL.
    c. Incorrect. A 30-day supply would only be 150 mL.
    d. Incorrect. A 10-day supply would only be 50 mL.

57. **Category I**

    a. Incorrect. This would supply the whole 20 mg.
    b. Incorrect. This would be 10 mg of Prozac.
    c. Incorrect. This would be 4 mg of Prozac.
    d. **Correct.** Use the ratio proportion method: x mL/1 mg = 5 mL/20 mg, x mL = 0.25 mL.

Chapter 4

58. **Category I**
    a. Incorrect. This is the answer if you use the wrong conversion of 1 in = 2 cm, when actually 1 in = 2.54 cm.
    b. Incorrect. This is miscalculating the number of inches in 5 ft, 2 in as only 60 in when it is 62 in.
    c. **Correct.** Note that 5 feet, 2 inches = 62 inches because there are 12 inches in 1 foot. Also, 1 inch = 2.54 cm. Using these figures, calculate the number of centimeters using the ratio-proportion method: x cm/62 inches = 2.54 cm/1 inch, x cm = 157.48 cm, rounded to 157.5 cm.
    d. Incorrect. This is the number of inches in 5 ft, 2 in.

59. **Category III**
    a. Incorrect. This is only the cost of the ingredients.
    b. Incorrect. This is the cost of ingredients and a 30% markup.
    c. Incorrect. This is the cost of ingredients and the compounding fee.
    d. **Correct.** First, calculate the markup: $8.76 × 0.3 = $2.63. Second, calculate the charge for the patient: $8.76 original price + $2.63 markup + $10.00 compounding fee = $21.39.

60. **Category III**
    a. Incorrect. This is when the insurer pays only for services rendered.
    b. **Correct.** Capitation is an amount of money paid per policy holder to a healthcare provider to provide all the needs that the patient has. If the patient does not need anything, then the provider made money; if the patient needs many services, then the fee may barely cover the cost or not at all.
    c. Incorrect. This is the manufacturer's estimated selling price for pharmaceuticals.
    d. Incorrect. This is the process of sending a claim via a modem to the insurer to verify payment.

61. **Category II**
    a. Incorrect. Although this is what you want, the wholesaler only sells the product in quantities of 10 vials at a time.
    b. **Correct.** Order the product that will bring you close to the maximum with a minimum of overage. Do not order a strength you do not normally carry.
    c. Incorrect. You need to order something, therefore you will not run out if you have another patient who needs Cytoxan.
    c. Incorrect. You do not stock this strength, and it will not replace what you used.

62. **Category II**
    a. Incorrect. Given that the turnover rate equals the annual dollars of purchase divided by average inventory value, this number is too small.
    b. **Correct.** Turnover rate = yearly purchases ÷ average inventory = $500,000.00 ÷ $125,000.00 = 4.
    c. Incorrect. Reversing the numbers produces this answer.
    d. Incorrect. Subtracting and reversing the numbers produces this answer.

63. **Category I**
    a. Incorrect. This is a drug that damages cellular DNA during replication.
    b. Incorrect. This drug binds irreversibly to DNA and stops replication.
    c. **Correct.** Leucovorin is given with methotrexate and fluorouracil to replenish active folic acid and decrease drug toxicity.
    d. Incorrect. This is a plant alkaloid that prevents the metaphase of cell division.

64. **Category I**
    a. **Correct.** The bone marrow produces red blood cells, and a drug that suppresses the bone marrow will decrease the number of red blood cells and cause anemia.
    b. Incorrect. This is an inflammation and ulceration of the mouth.

c. Incorrect. This is the other name for hair loss.

d. Incorrect. This is also a result of bone marrow suppression, but it is a loss of white blood cells and increases a patient's risk of infection.

65. Category I

a. Incorrect. Thiazide diuretics cause potassium wasting by the kidneys.

b. **Correct.** Triamterene, amiloride, and spironolactone are the three potassium-sparing diuretics available.

c. Incorrect. Metolazone works similar to thiazide diuretics and leads to potassium loss.

d. Incorrect. Furosemide is a loop diuretic and causes an increase in potassium loss.

66. Category I

a. Incorrect. Aciphex (rabeprazole) is a proton pump inhibitor used to treat ulcers.

b. Incorrect. Accutane (isotretinoin) is an agent used to treat acne.

c. Incorrect. Accupril (quinapril) is an ACE inhibitor used to treat hypertension.

d. **Correct.** Aricept (donepezil) was one of the first agents approved to slow the process of Alzheimer's disease.

67. Category I

a. Incorrect. Never make a statement that requires professional judgment; always offer to have the pharmacist explain in these situations.

b. **Correct.** Given that this question requires professional judgment, the pharmacist should be called to explain to the patient.

c. Incorrect. A pharmacy technician should always have the pharmacist explain about drug indications and reasons for taking a particular medication.

d. Incorrect. Never say anyone has made a mistake. Offer to look into it, and notify the pharmacist.

68. Category I

a. **Correct.** Eye contact is a nonverbal form of communication indicating that you have my attention.

b. Incorrect. Empathy is relating back to what someone has just said and your understanding of how he or she feels.

c. Incorrect. Even talking softly is verbal communication.

d. Incorrect. Calling people by a respectful title, such as Doctor or Mrs., is again verbal communication.

69. Category I

a. Incorrect. No part of the capsule is called the top.

b. Incorrect. No part of the capsule is called the bottom.

c. **Correct.** The body is used to punch the powder, and the cap is placed on the body to hold the powder in.

d. Incorrect. The cap covers the body once it is *punched* with powder.

70. Category I

a. Incorrect. This is the largest capsule size.

b. Incorrect. This is the third from the largest capsule size.

c. Incorrect. This is the fourth from the largest capsule size.

d. **Correct.** The larger the number is, the smaller the capsule will be, with 000 being the largest.

71. Category I

a. Incorrect. This will make a very coarse powder.

b. Incorrect. This will make a coarse powder.

c. Incorrect. This will make a fine powder.

d. **Correct.** The higher the sieve number is, the finer the powder that can be shaken through it will be.

72. Category I

a. Incorrect. This is a solution made with alcohol.

b. **Correct.** A suspension is a dispersion of a solid or oil in a liquid vehicle.

c. Incorrect. The active ingredient is dissolved in the vehicle.

d. Incorrect. The active ingredient is dissolved in the vehicle.

73. Category II

a. **Correct.** Good manufacturing practices are the guidelines that pharmacists and manufacturers must follow to guarantee that a product is compounded appropriately.

b. Incorrect. This is a fictitious answer.

c. Incorrect. Manufacturing is not done in pharmacies but by manufacturers.

d. Incorrect. This is a fictitious answer.

74. Category I

a. Incorrect. At present, no vaccine has been produced to prevent HIV.

b. Incorrect. At present, no vaccine has been produced for herpes simplex.

c. **Correct.** Once a year, high-risk populations and healthcare professionals get vaccinated against the influenza virus.

d. Incorrect. At present, no vaccine has been produced for cytomegalovirus.

75. Category II

a. Incorrect. Morphine is not the drug of choice for narcotic addiction.

b. Incorrect. Naloxone blocks opioid receptors, causing immediate withdrawal and is therefore not used for narcotic addiction but for overdose.

c. Incorrect. Butorphanol is a narcotic agonist-antagonist used to treat pain.

d. **Correct.** Methadone for maintenance and detoxification from heroin or other opioids may only be dispensed at specially DEA-licensed sites.

76. Category I

a. Incorrect. This is a self-administered test to monitor signs and symptoms of depression.

b. Incorrect. Renal function is not monitored weekly in these patients.

c. **Correct.** Also called leukocytes, the white blood cell count must be checked regularly in patients on Clozaril because a major side effect of this drug is agranulocytosis, and patients die from the inability to fight infections.

d. Incorrect. Red blood cell count is tested for anemia, and Clozaril does not regularly cause anemia.

77. Category I

a. **Correct.** BuSpar (buspirone) is not a controlled substance but does require a prescription.

b. Incorrect. This is a class-IV agent.

c. Incorrect. This is a class-IV agent.

d. Incorrect. This is a class-IV agent.

78. Category I

a. Incorrect. Drugs such as cephalexin and cefazolin are first-generation drugs.

b. Incorrect. Drugs such as cefaclor and cefoxitin are second-generation drugs.

c. Incorrect. Drugs such as ceftriaxone and cefditoren are third-generation drugs.

d. **Correct.** Cefepime is a fourth-generation cephalosporin, with activity against gram-negative rods.

79. Category I

a. Incorrect. Erythromycin is a macrolide, and gentamicin is an aminoglycoside.

b. **Correct.** Biaxin (clarithromycin) is also a macrolide, similar to erythromycin, and should be avoided in this patient.

c. Incorrect. Penicillin should be fine if erythromycin is her only allergy medication.

d. Incorrect. Doxycycline is a tetracycline and should be fine if erythromycin is her only allergy medication.

Chapter 4

80. Category I

a. Incorrect. This is the trade name that is used exclusively by the manufacturer of the drug.
b. Incorrect. This is the name that describes the chemical composition of the active ingredient.
c. **Correct.** The generic name is the USAN name.
d. Incorrect. The drug is patented by the pharmaceutical research company; therefore no one can take the idea and develop the drug first.

81. Category I

a. **Correct.** As directed in USP 797, working in a hood requires working at least 6 in from all edges.
b. Incorrect. You would be too close to the high-efficiency particulate air (HEPA) filter and straining your arms.
c. Incorrect. You would be too close to the HEPA filter and straining your arms.
d. Incorrect. You are working too far away, which may result in contamination.

82. Category I

a. Incorrect. This is the amount of sterile water you would need to make the final product.
b. Incorrect. Misinterpreting the 0.8% as 0.008 g in 100 mL would produce this answer.
c. **Correct.** Using alligation solve the problem:

10		0.8 mL parts 10%
	0.8	
0		9.2 mL parts 0%
		10 mL total parts 0.8%

x mL/500 mL = 0.8 mL parts 10%/ 10 mL total parts, x mL = 40 mL 10%
x mL/500 mL = 9.2 mL parts 0%/ 10 mL total parts, x mL = 460 mL 0% (sterile water)
d. Incorrect. Misinterpreting both percentage numbers would produce this answer.

83. Category I

a. Incorrect. Instead of 10 mEq, you used 7.5 mEq.
b. **Correct.** Add the atomic weights of each element in KCl: 39.1 + 35.5 = 74.6. This number equals the number of 1 mEq of KCl. Therefore, this number multiplied by 10 equals the number of milligrams per milliliter in 10 mEq KCl: 74.6 × 10 = 746 mg/mL.
c. Incorrect. This is only the weight of the potassium taken into consideration.
d. Incorrect. This is only the weight of the chloride taken into consideration.

84. Category I

a. **Correct.** Penicillin in the injectable form is still measured in units.
b. Incorrect. Warfarin is measured in milligrams.
c. Incorrect. Esmolol is measured in milligrams.
d. Incorrect. Cyanocobolamine is measured in micrograms.

85. Category I

a. Incorrect. The use of the drug is included in the package insert.
b. Incorrect. The precautions pertaining to the drug are in the package insert.
c. Incorrect. The revision date is in the package insert.
d. **Correct.** The package insert does not have any information about cost.

Chapter 4

86. Category III

a. Incorrect. The director of pharmacy reports to someone such as a vice president in charge of professional services.
b. **Correct.** The president or chief executive officer (CEO) reports to the board of directors.
c. Incorrect. This person reports to the president.
d. Incorrect. Staff pharmacists usually report to the director of pharmacy, as would the pharmacy technicians.

87. Category III

  a. Incorrect. Only a registered pharmacist may perform this duty.

  b. Incorrect. Only a registered pharmacist may receive a verbal order.

  c. **Correct.** A pharmacy technician may take a written prescription from a patient for processing.

  d. Incorrect. The pharmacist is responsible for verification.

88. Category II

  a. Incorrect. HIPAA requires the patient to be notified and to authorize any sale of medical information.

  b. **Correct.** HIPAA establishes a law that only permits the patient to give permission for release of personal health information.

  c. Incorrect. The intellectual property contained in the medical record is the patient's but not the medical record itself.

  d. Incorrect. A patient may request a copy of his or her medical record without a court order.

89. Category III

  a. **Correct.** A nuclear pharmacy compounds radiopharmaceuticals for diagnostic and therapeutic use.

  b. Incorrect. This is the area that applies the pharmacist's knowledge.

  c. Incorrect. This is another name for a retail pharmacy.

  d. Incorrect. This refers to a pharmacy in an institution such as a hospital or psychiatric facility.

90. Category I

  a. Incorrect. The patient's name must be on the prescription.

  b. Incorrect. The date written should be on a prescription.

  c. **Correct.** The responsible party for payment is needed by the pharmacy and must be gathered from the patient, but this information is not on the prescription.

  d. Incorrect. Refill information should be included or assumed as *no refills* if not filled in.

91. Category I

  a. **Correct.** A prescriber's DEA number must be on a prescription for a controlled substance only.

  b. Incorrect. Only written prescriptions must have the physician's actual signature.

  c. Incorrect. This should be on all prescriptions to help locate the physician in case of questions.

  d. Incorrect. The date written should be on all prescriptions.

92. Category II

  a. Incorrect. Aseptic technique is used to compound sterile products.

  b. **Correct.** Wiping the counting tray prevents cross-contamination of drug products.

  c. Incorrect. Counter washing is good for cleanliness but does not stop cross-contamination.

  d. Incorrect. Latex gloves or any gloves are not used in filling solid dose form prescriptions.

93. Category I

  a. Incorrect. This is the legally required auxiliary label to be attached to all controlled substances.

  b. Incorrect. Although antibiotics can cause failure of birth control pills, this is not the reason for resistance.

  c. **Correct.** Patients not completing a course of antibiotics may lead to resistance.

  d. Incorrect. Food may decrease absorption of some antibiotics, but it is not one of the mechanisms of resistance.

94. Category I

  a. **Correct.** Amphotericin B should only be mixed in dextrose or it will precipitate.

  b. Incorrect. Amphotericin B should only be mixed in dextrose or it will precipitate.

Chapter 4

c. Incorrect. Amphotericin B should only be mixed in dextrose or it will precipitate.
d. Incorrect. Amphotericin B should only be mixed in dextrose or it will precipitate.

95. Category II

a. Incorrect. This is a patch that gradually releases the drug at a controlled rate over a specific period.
b. Incorrect. This is a parenteral injection that must be administered by a nurse.
c. **Correct.** Patient-controlled analgesia is a method of pain relief that actually uses less narcotic because the patient can dose him or herself early in the management of pain and not have to wait for a nurse.
d. Incorrect. This is a catheter placed near the spine to control pain.

96. Category II

a. Incorrect. This is used to order class-II drugs.
b. Incorrect. This is a triplicate form.
c. **Correct.** Only one item may be ordered per line.
d. Incorrect. Only an employee with power of attorney may sign the form.

97. Category II

a. **Correct.** Proper storage of medication is necessary to guarantee the safety and efficacy of a drug.
b. Incorrect. Checking the refrigerator temperature is a quality-assurance technique that allows proof that drugs are stored at the appropriate temperature and that the inventory is not being wasted by improper storage.
c. Incorrect. Although a repackaged product may need to be refrigerated, the temperature is checked for quality assurance.
d. Incorrect. The five rights are patient, drug, strength, route, and time.

98. Category I

a. Incorrect. Adding sodium chloride with calcium gluconate is not a problem.
b. Incorrect. Adding potassium chloride with calcium gluconate is not a problem.
c. Incorrect. Adding magnesium sulfate with calcium gluconate is not a problem.
d. **Correct.** Potassium phosphate and calcium gluconate, when added together or in an excessively high concentration, will form an insoluble precipitate.

99. Category III

a. Incorrect. The hood should be on at all times. If it is turned off, it should run 30 minutes before use.
b. **Correct.** A hood must be cleaned at the beginning of the day and repeatedly throughout the day to ensure a clean environment in which to prepare sterile products.
c. Incorrect. Air currents may contaminate the hood working area.
d. Incorrect. Necessary materials to mix should be wiped with alcohol and placed in the hood so you do not have to leave the hood once you start mixing.

100. Category I

a. Incorrect. This is a medicine for insomnia and would not be used in the morning.
b. Incorrect. This medication is only taken once a day at bedtime.
c. Incorrect. This medication is only taken once a day at bedtime.
d. **Correct.** Ambien (zolpidem) is a hypnotic and is given to induce sleep.

101. Category I

a. Incorrect. This insulin is short acting and injected subcutaneously right before meals.

Chapter 4

b. Incorrect. This insulin is long acting and is a suspension that can only be injected subcutaneously.

c. Incorrect. This is long acting with no noticeable peak and must be injected subcutaneously to work properly.

d. **Correct.** Only regular insulin may be administered IV.

102. Category I

a. Incorrect. This is a question requiring professional judgment and should be referred to the pharmacist.

b. Incorrect. The technician may look up a dose and give the information to the pharmacist but may not give the answer directly to the physician.

c. Incorrect. Another technician would only be able to help you turn the question over to a pharmacist.

d. **Correct.** Pharmacy technicians should always refer professional judgment questions about a drug to the pharmacist.

103. Category II

a. Incorrect. ISMP and JCAHO have banned the use of trailing zeros.

b. **Correct.** Do not include any trailing zeros, unnecessary decimal points, or leading zeros that may confuse the order.

c. Incorrect. This is only one half of one milligram.

d. Incorrect. Although this is another way of writing 5 mg, it is not the best answer to this question.

104. Category I

a. Incorrect. This is not a solid dose form, therefore the verb *take* is inappropriate.

b. Incorrect. This needs more information to be correct.

c. **Correct.** The Serevent Diskus is a device that is breath activated, and the medication is inhaled into the lungs. Directions would be *inhale one puff by mouth two times a day*.

d. Incorrect. This is an inhaler, not a capsule.

105. Category I

a. Incorrect. This machine is used to stock medications on patient care areas for use by the nursing staff for patient orders.

b. Incorrect. This is a delivery system used in larger hospitals to deliver medications from the pharmacy to the patient care area.

c. Incorrect. This is an IV set that is used to administer medications.

d. **Correct.** When compounding numerous, large-volume parenteral medications in a day, larger pharmacies use a machine such as the Micromix admixture compounder to make the process more efficient.

106. Category I

a. Incorrect. This requires years of education as attained by a pharmacist in college, but it is not necessary as part of appropriate communication techniques.

b. **Correct.** Not only being able to talk effectively, but also being able to listen and interpret others is important.

c. Incorrect. You can communicate effectively on the telephone without eye contact.

d. Incorrect. Although this is a nice quality, it is not necessary for communicating effectively.

107. Category I

a. Incorrect. This risk level means no risk in pregnancy.

b. Incorrect. This risk level means caution is advised.

c. **Correct.** A pregnancy risk of *D* indicates that human or animal studies have identified a definite risk.

d. Incorrect. This risk level means these drugs are not to be used in pregnancy.

108. Category II

a. Incorrect. This is purchasing pharmaceuticals from each individual manufacturer.

b. **Correct.** A wholesaler is a "middle-man" that provides pharmaceuticals at a contracted price to a pharmacy from various sources.

c. Incorrect. This is the mechanism of ordering medications in quantities in time to meet demand.

d. Incorrect. This is purchasing products that are not available through group purchasing, such as specialty products.

109. Category I

a. Incorrect. This amendment to the FDCA establishes the difference between prescription and OTC medications.

b. **Correct.** The Drug Listing Act developed the NDC to enable the FDA to have a listing of all approved drug products in the United States.

c. Incorrect. This Act prevents reimportation of pharmaceuticals from foreign countries.

d. Incorrect. HIPAA is the Act that allows you to keep insurance when you leave a job, as outlined in the Consolidated Omnibus Budget Reconciliation Act of 1985 (COBRA), and makes healthcare individuals and organizations accountable for the confidentiality of patient healthcare information.

110. Category I

a. Incorrect. Antihistamines do not cause a rebound rhinitis.

b. Incorrect. Cough suppressants do not cause a rebound-rhinitis.

c. Incorrect. Agents that lower blood pressure do not cause a rebound rhinitis.

d. **Correct.** Nasal decongestants should not be used for longer than 3 days at recommended doses.

111. Category I

a. Incorrect. Dairy products do not affect the absorption of metronidazole.

b. Incorrect. Metronidazole does not cause drowsiness.

c. Incorrect. You do not have to avoid sunlight while taking metronidazole.

d. **Correct.** The combination of Flagyl (metronidazole) with alcohol will result in a disulfiram-like reaction in which the patient will feel lightheaded and nauseous.

112. Category III

a. **Correct.** A nosocomial infection is acquired while a patient is in a medical facility.

b. Incorrect. Empiric therapy means treating without knowing the causative agent.

c. Incorrect. This is a term for a bacterium that needs oxygen to survive.

d. Incorrect. This is a new infection that complicates the course of therapy for an existing infection.

113. Category II

a. Incorrect. The FDA enforces manufacturing regulations.

b. Incorrect. This group enforces the Poison Prevention Act.

c. **Correct.** Under the Controlled Substance Act, the DEA is responsible for enforcing the law pertaining to controlled substances.

d. Incorrect. HIPAA violations can be reported to this group.

114. Category I

Chapter 4

a. Incorrect. Although gout is painful and acetaminophen (Tylenol) is a pain reliever, it does not treat gout.

b. Incorrect. Acetazolamide (Diamox) is a diuretic that is used to decrease intraocular pressure of glaucoma.

c. Incorrect. Acarbose (Precose) is an agent that prevents absorption of carbohydrates and is used to control blood sugar.

d. **Correct.** Allopurinol (Zyloprim) is one of the agents used to manage gout.

115. Category II

a. Incorrect. Turnover is how often you sell the value of your inventory.
b. **Correct.** More receipts means more money was taken in (income) than was paid out (expenses), also known as profit.
c. Incorrect. This is the difference between an item's cost to the pharmacy and its selling price to patients.
d. Incorrect. This is a charge to the patient that takes into account overhead and professional costs of dispensing the prescription.

116. Category II

a. **Correct.** If a drug is contaminated in the manufacturing process or storage, a recall may be issued.
b. Incorrect. A manufacturer may stop production of a drug because of low profit, but a recall involves adverse effects, not profits.
c. Incorrect. A notification may be disseminated for a label change, but this is not a reason to recall a drug unless it is labeled wrong and leads to adverse reactions.
d. Incorrect. Advertising is not involved in recalls.

117. Category II

a. Incorrect. When receiving, the name of the product is one of the first things to check, which ensures that you received the right product.
b. Incorrect. Many drugs are available in a variety of strengths, and you need to make sure you receive the one you ordered.
c. Incorrect. Make sure you received the amount for which you were charged.
d. **Correct.** Cost is not part of the receiving process, but it should be checked against the contracted price to make sure the pharmacy is not overcharged.

118. Category II

a. Incorrect. The idea is to place short-dated products where they will be used first, therefore placing the item in the back of other stock is not ideal.
b. Incorrect. This will only clutter the work space.
c. **Correct.** When stocking shelves, always rotate the stock, and make sure the product with the shortest dating is in front so as to be used first.
d. Incorrect. This will not allow easy identification of stock that should be used first.

119. Category I

a. Incorrect. Using the apothecary-metric conversion, 1 fl oz = 30 mL, this answer is only 15 mL.
b. **Correct.** Know the conversion 1 fl oz = 30 mL.
c. Incorrect. This would be 60 mL.
d. Incorrect. This would be 120 mL.

120. Category I

a. Incorrect. This is a metric measure of volume.
b. Incorrect. This is a metric measure of weight.
c. Incorrect. This is a household measure of volume.
d. **Correct.** A grain is a unit of weight in the apothecary system.

121. Category II

a. Incorrect. This is not a reason to take a drug off formulary.
b. **Correct.** Many products are not available in unit doses, therefore the technician will have to repackage the drug in the appropriate unit-dose packaging.
c. Incorrect. To prevent medication errors, bulk packages are not sent to the patient care area.
d. Incorrect. Only the P&T committee may make a therapeutic change to formulary.

122. **Category II**

    a. **Correct.** Cephalexin pediatric suspension should be refrigerated and shaken before use.

    b. Incorrect. This formulation does not need to be refrigerated.

    c. Incorrect. This formulation does not need to be refrigerated.

    d. Incorrect. This formulation does not need to be refrigerated.

123. **Category III**

    a. Incorrect. This book would contain information on products that are extemporaneously compounded.

    b. Incorrect. This log is a list of products that have been unit dosed.

    c. **Correct.** Always check the policy and procedure manual for information on the appropriate handling of drug products.

    d. Incorrect. This manual usually contains job descriptions, hiring information, and similar information in which human resources might be involved.

124. **Category III**

    a. Incorrect. This is a process of collecting names on a list with a commonality.

    b. Incorrect. Licensure is a process required to practice a profession.

    c. Incorrect. Voluntarily taking an examination to demonstrate proficiency is certification.

    d. **Correct.** Institutions such as hospitals undergo inspection for accreditation to prove that they meet a certain level of care.

125. **Category I**

    a. Incorrect. Failing to convert pounds to kilograms produces this answer.

    b. **Correct.** First, calculate the patient's weight in kilograms: 210 lb $\times$ 1 kg/2.2 lb = 95.454 kg, rounded to 95.5 kg. Second, calculate the dose per hour: 95.5 kg $\times$ 10 units/kg/hr = 955 units/hr. Third, use the ratio-proportion method to calculate the volume of the stock solution that will provide this rate: x mL/955 units = 500 mL/25,000 units, x mL = 19.1 mL/hr.

    c. Incorrect. Assuming that the stock solution is 25,000 units/L produces this answer.

    d. Incorrect. Using the incorrect dose of 1 unit/kg/hr produces this answer.

126. **Category I**

    a. Incorrect. Changes in insurance coverage affect payment and must be updated regularly.

    b. Incorrect. Many OTC medications can adversely affect prescription medications, and knowing this information can prevent drug interactions.

    c. Incorrect. Always ask about allergy information because it may change with time.

    d. **Correct.** Addiction history may not be something about which the patient is comfortable talking and is not required for updating a profile by a technician.

127. **Category I**

    a. Incorrect. This is the number of days the patient will be on the therapy.

    b. Incorrect. This number is correct if the patient were on each daily schedule for 4 days. However, after 8 days, the daily schedule drops to 2 days of therapy.

    c. **Correct.** Add up the total number of doses (16 + 12 + 4 + 2 + 1 = 35).

    d. Incorrect. If you do not split the tablet on the last 2 days and save the half tablet, you might need an extra tablet, but pharmacies do not usually give extras this way.

Chapter 4

128. **Category I**
   a. Incorrect. This is the abbreviation for eye drops, and Patanol is used to treat allergic eye symptoms.
   b. **Correct.** Although *ou* is not an acceptable abbreviation, many physicians still write it, and you need to know it means *both eyes*.
   c. Incorrect. The abbreviation for the right eye is *od*.
   d. Incorrect. The abbreviation for the right ear is *ad*.

129. **Category I**
   a. **Correct.** Given that the patient is a woman, she would not need a drug for benign prostate hyperplasia; women do not have prostates.
   b. Incorrect. ProSom is not an estrogen product.
   c. Incorrect. Both men and women can take ProSom, therefore this is not the best answer to the question.
   d. Incorrect. Proscar is taken once a day, therefore this does not help answer the question.

130. **Category II**
   a. Incorrect. Hormone replacement therapy is not exempt from child-resistant packaging.
   b. **Correct.** Given that these are dispensed in the manufacturer-provided monthly packets, they do not need to be in a child-resistant container.
   c. Incorrect. ISDN sublingual and chewable is exempt but not isosorbide mononitrate.
   d. Incorrect. Unit-dose forms of potassium chloride are available in packets of powder or effervescent tablets but not oral tablets.

131. **Category II**
   a. Incorrect. Once the patient is using the drug, it may be stored at room temperature.
   b. Incorrect. Freezing may alter the drug.
   c. Incorrect. This is not a controlled substance.
   d. **Correct.** The package label on Xalatan indicates that it should be refrigerated until dispensed.

132. **Category I**
   a. Incorrect. This is the act of combining two substances.
   b. **Correct.** Comminution is the act of reducing a substance to a small, fine, particle-like talc for body powder.
   c. Incorrect. This is the process of grinding.
   d. Incorrect. This is the technique to incorporate materials into an ointment.

133. **Category II**
   a. Incorrect. A formulary list or want book would help with purchasing.
   b. Incorrect. A markup formula would help with pricing.
   c. **Correct.** Extemporaneous compounding should be documented on a master formula sheet.
   d. Incorrect. A policy and procedure manual would help with this.

134. **Category I**
   a. **Correct.** Lactose is a diluent used in making tablets and capsules.
   b. Incorrect. This is used to make suppositories.
   c. Incorrect. This is used to make suppositories.
   d. Incorrect. This is used to make suppositories.

135. **Category I**
   a. Incorrect. This is not a therapeutic use of a radionuclide.
   b. **Correct.** A radioactive form of iodine (I-131) is used to treat hyperthyroidism.
   c. Incorrect. This is treated with thyroid replacement.
   d. Incorrect. A radionuclide is not needed to x-ray for broken bones.

Chapter 4

136. Category II

a. Incorrect. NABP has no regulatory authority.
b. Incorrect. The FDA has authority over manufacturing.
c. Incorrect. The DEA only has authority over controlled substances.
d. **Correct.** Each state has the sole regulatory oversight for the practice of pharmacies in that state.

137. Category II

a. Incorrect. The FDA does not have authority over the nutritional supplement market.
b. **Correct.** This Act sets a limitation on the activity that the FDA can have on the dietary supplement market. Most individuals do not realize that the FDA's rigorous approval process is not used for dietary supplements.
c. Incorrect. Manufacturers of supplements may not make health claims, only that they can be used to support health.
d. Incorrect. If the FDA wants to remove a nutritional supplement, it must prove that it is unsafe.

138. Category I

a. Incorrect. This is the brand name of alprazolam.
b. Incorrect. This is the brand name of ranitidine.
c. **Correct.** Xeloda is the brand name for capecitabine, an oral antineoplastic that the body converts to fluorouracil.
d. Incorrect. This is the brand name of goserelin.

139. Category I

a. **Correct.** Calculate the number of tablets using the ratio-proportion method: x tablets/$10 = 100 tablets/$29.79, x tablets = 33.568 tablets, rounded down to 33 tablets (or $.30/tablet $\times$ 33 tablets = $9.90).
b. Incorrect. This would short the buyer three tablets.
c. Incorrect. This would give him too many tablets, and you would lose profit.
d. Incorrect. Patients are allowed to fill prescriptions partially and should be accommodated.

140. Category I

a. Incorrect. This is a substance that kills bacteria.
b. Incorrect. This means to remove infectious agents from objects.
c. Incorrect. This means free of infection or contamination.
d. **Correct.** The suffix -*stasis* means *to stop* or *inhibit*, therefore bacteriostatic means to inhibit growth of bacteria.

Chapter 4

Common Prescription Abbreviations and Unsafe Abbreviations

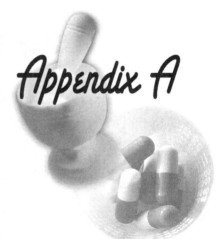

Appendix A

Abbreviations Used in Writing Prescriptions

Abbreviation	Translation
ac	before meals
bid	twice a day
c	with
cap	capsule
DAW	dispense as written
D/C	discontinue
g	gram*
gr	grain
gtt	drop
hs	at bedtime
IM	intramuscular
IV	intravenously
L	liter
mcg	microgram
mEq	milliequivalent
mL	milliliter
NKA	no known allergy
NKDA	no known drug allergy
npo	nothing by mouth
pc	after meals
po	by mouth
prn	as needed
q	every
qh	every hour
q2h	every 2 hours
qid	four times a day
qs	a sufficient quantity
stat	immediately
tab	tablet
tid	three times daily
ud	as directed
wk	week

* The abbreviation *gm* is sometimes used for *gram*.

Note: Some prescribers may write abbreviations using capital letters or periods. However, periods should not be used with metrics or medical abbreviations as they can be a source of medication errors.

Problematic Prescription Abbreviations

Unapproved Abbreviation	Correct Form to Use
mg	microgram or mcg
qd	every day
qod	every other day
U	units
MgSO4	magnesium sulfate
MSO4	morphine sulfate
no leading zero, .2 (often read as 2, creating a tenfold error)	0.2
Trailing zero, 2.0 (often read as 20, creating a tenfold error)	2

Note: Additional dangerous abbreviations are listed at www.ismp.org.

Guide for Preventing Prescription Errors

Appendix B

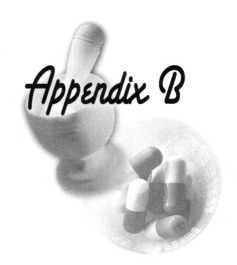

While manufacturers have an obligation to review new trademarks for error potential before use, there are some things that prescribers, pharmacists, and pharmacy technicians can do to help prevent errors with products that have look- or sound-alike names. The Institute for Safe Medication Practices (ISMP) (www.ismp.org) has provided following recommendations designed to prevent dispensing errors.

- **Use electronic prescribing** to prevent confusion with handwritten drug names.
- **Encourage physicians to write prescriptions that clearly specify the dosage form, drug strength, and complete directions.** They should include the product's indication on all outpatient prescriptions and on inpatient *prn* orders. With name pairs known to be problematic, reduce the potential for confusion by writing prescriptions using both the brand and generic name. Listing both names on medication administration records and automated dispensing cabinet computer screens also may be helpful.
- **Whenever possible, determine the purpose of the medication** before dispensing or administering it. Many products with look-alike or sound-alike names are used for different purposes.
- **Accept verbal or telephone orders only when truly necessary.** Require staff to read back all orders, spell the product name, and state its indication. Like medication names, numbers can sound alike, so staff should read the dosage back in numerals (e.g., "one five" for fifteen milligrams) to ensure clear interpretation of dose.

- **When feasible, use magnifying lenses and copyholders** under good lighting to keep prescriptions and orders at eye level during transcription to improve the likelihood of proper interpretation of look-alike product names.
- **Change the appearance of look-alike product names** on computer screens, pharmacy and nursing unit shelf labels, and bins (including automated dispensing cabinets), pharmacy product labels, and medication administration records by highlighting, through boldface, color, and/or tall man letters, the parts of the names that are different (e.g., hydrOXYzine, hydrALAzine).
- **Install a computerized reminder** (also placed on automated dispensing cabinet screens) for the most serious confusing name pairs so that an alert is generated when entering prescriptions for either drug. If possible, make the reminder auditory as well as visual.
- **Affix "name alert" stickers** in areas where look-alike or sound-alike products are stored (available from pharmacy label manufacturers).
- **Store products with look-alike or sound-alike names in different locations**. Avoid storing both products in the fast-mover area. Use a shelf sticker to help locate the product that is moved.
- **Continue to employ an independent check in the dispensing process** (one person interprets and enters the prescription into the computer and another reviews the printed label against the original prescription and the product).
- **Open the prescription bottle or the unit dose package in front of the patient** to confirm the expected product appearance and review the indication. Caution patients about error potential when taking products that have a look-alike or sound-alike counterpart. Take the time to fully investigate the situation if a patient states he or she is taking an unknown medication.
- **Monitor reported errors caused by look-alike and sound-alike medication names** and alert staff to mistakes.
- **Look for the possibility of name confusion when a new product is added to the formulary.** Have a few clinicians handwrite the product name and directions, as they would appear in a typical order. Ask front-line nurses, pharmacists, technicians, unit secretaries, and physicians to view the samples of the written product name as well as pronounce it to determine if it looks or sounds like any other drug product or medical term. It may be helpful to have clinicians first look at the scripted product name to determine how they would interpret it before the actual product name is provided to them for pronunciation. Once the product name is known, clinicians may be less likely to see more familiar product names in the written samples. If the potential for confusion with other products is identified, take steps to avoid errors as listed in the points that follow.

- **Encourage reporting of errors** and potentially hazardous conditions with look-alike and sound-alike product names and use the information to establish priorities for error reduction. Also maintain awareness of problematic product names and error prevention recommendations provided by ISMP (www.ismp.org and also listed on the quarterly *Action Agenda*), FDA (www.fda.gov), and USP (www.usp.org).
- **Review Table B.1 for look-alike and sound-alike drug name pairs in use at your practice location.** Decide what actions might be warranted to prevent medication errors. Stay current with alerts from ISMP, FDA, and USP in case new problematic name pairs emerge.

Table B.1 Look-Alike and Sound-Alike Medications

Abelcet	amphotericin B	
Accupril	Aciphex	
acetazolamide	acetohexamide	
acetohexamide	acetazolamide	
Aciphex	Aricept	
Aciphex	Accupril	
Activase	TNKase	
Actonel	Actos	
Actos	Actonel	
Adderall	Inderal	
Advicor	Altocor	
Aggrastat	argatroban	
Aldara	Alora	
Alkeran	Leukeran	Myleran
Allegra	Viagra	
Alora	Aldara	
Altocor	Advicor	
Amaryl	Reminyl	
AmBisome	amphotericin B	
amphotericin B	Abelcet	
amphotericin B	Ambisome	
antacid	Atacand	
Antivert	Axert	
Anzemet	Avandamet	
argatroban	Aggrastat	
Aricept	Aciphex	
aripiprazole	proton pump inhibitors	
aripiprazole	rabeprazole	
Asacol	Os-Cal	
Atacand	antacid	
Atrovent	Natru-Vent	
Avandamet	Anzemet	
Avandia	Prandin	
Avandia	Coumadin	
Avinza	Invanz	
Avinza	Evista	

Continues

Table B.1 Look-Alike and Sound-Alike Medications—*continued*

Axert	Antivert	
BayHep B	BayRab	BayRho-D
BayRab	BayRho-D	BayHep B
BayRho-D	BayHep B	BayRab
Bicillin C-R	Bicillin L-A	
Bicillin L-A	Bicillin C-R	
Brethine	Methergine	
camphorated tincture of opium (paregoric)	opium tincture	
carboplatin	cisplatin	
Cedax	Cidex	
Celexa	Zyprexa	
chlorpromazine	chlorpropamide	
chlorpropamide	chlorpromazine	
Cidex	Cedax	
cisplatin	carboplatin	
Claritin-D	Claritin-D 24	
Claritin-D 24	Claritin-D	
Clozaril	Colazal	
Colace	Cozaar	
Colazal	Clozaril	
colchicine	Cortrosyn	
Comvax	Recombivax HB	
Cortrosyn	colchicine	
Coumadin	Avandia	
Cozaar	Colace	
Cozaar	Zocor	
dactinomycin	daptomycin	
daptomycin	dactinomycin	
Darvon	Diovan	
daunorubicin	idarubicin	
Denavir	Indinavir	
Depakote	Depakote ER	
Depakote ER	Depakote	
Depo-Medrol	Solu-Medrol	
Diabenese	Diamox	
DiaBeta	Zebeta	
Diamox	Diabenese	
Diatex (diazepam in Mexico)	Diatx	
Diatx	Diatex (diazepam in Mexico)	
Dilacor XR	Pilocar	
Dilaudid	Dilaudid-5	
Dilaudid-5	Dilaudid	
Dioval	Diovan	
Diovan	Dioval	
Diovan	Zyban	
Diovan	Darvon	
Diprivan	Ditropan	
Ditropan	Diprivan	
dobutamine	dopamine	

Table B.1 Look-Alike and Sound-Alike Medications—*continued*

dopamine	dobutamine
doxorubicin hydrochloride	liposomal doxorubicin (Doxil)
Duricef	Ultracet
Enbrel	Levbid
Endocet	Indocin
Engerix-B adult	Engerix-B pediatric/adolescent
Engerix-B pediatric/adolescent	Engerix-B adult
ephedrine	epinephrine
epinephrine	ephedrine
Estratest	Estratest H.S.
Estratest H.S.	Estratest
ethambutol	Ethmozine
Ethmozine	ethambutol
Evista	Avinza
Femara	Femhrt
Femhrt	Femara
fentanyl	sufentanil
folic acid	folinic acid (leucovorin calcium)
folinic acid (leucovorin calcium)	folic acid
Foradil	Toradol
gentamicin	gentian violet
gentian violet	gentamicin
Granulex	Regranex
Healon	Hyalgan
heparin	Hespan
Hespan	heparin
Humalog	Humulin
Humalog Mix 75/25	Humulin 70/30
Humulin	Humalog
Humulin 70/30	Humalog Mix 75/25
Hyalgan	Healon
hydromorphone	morphine
idarubicin	daunorubicin
Inderal	Adderall
indinavir	Denavir
Indocin	Endocet
infliximab	rituximab
Invanz	Avinza
iodine	Lodine
Isordil	Plendil
isotretinoin	tretinoin
K-Phos Neutral	Neutra-Phos K
Kaletra	Keppra
Keppra	Kaletra
Ketalar	ketorolac
ketorolac	Ketalar
Lamictal	Lamisil
Lamisil	Lamictal
lamivudine	lamotrigine
lamotrigine	lamivudine

Continues

Table B.1 Look-Alike and Sound-Alike Medications—*continued*

Lanoxin	levothyroxine	
Lantus	Lente	
Lasix	Luvox	
Lente	Lantus	
leucovorin calcium	Leukeran	
Leukeran	Myleran	Alkeran
Levbid	Enbrel	
levothyroxine	Lanoxin	
Lexapro	Loxitane	
Lipitor	Zyrtec	
liposomal doxorubicin (Doxil)	doxorubicin hydrochloride	
Lodine	iodine	
Lotronex	Protonix	
Loxitane	Lexapro	
Lupron Depot-3 Month	Lupron Depot-Ped	
Lupron Depot-Ped	Lupron Depot-3 Month	
Luvox	Lasix	
Maxzide	Microzide	
Metadate	methadone	
Metadate CD	Metadate ER	
Metadate ER	Metadate CD	
Metadate ER	methadone	
methadone	Metadate ER	
methadone	Metadate	
Methergine	Brethine	
Micronase	Microzide	
Microzide	Maxzide	
Microzide	Micronase	
mifepristone	misoprostol	
Miralax	Mirapex	
Mirapex	Miralax	
misoprostol	mifepristone	
morphine	hydromorphone	
morphine, oral liquid concentrate	morphine, non-concentrated oral liquid	
MS Contin	OxyContin	
Mucinex	Mucomyst	
Mucomyst	Mucinex	
Myleran	Alkeran	Leukeran
Narcan	Norcuron	
Natru-Vent	Atrovent	
Navane	Norvasc	
Neulasta	Neumega	
Neumega	Neupogen	
Neumega	Neulasta	
Neupogen	Neumega	
Neurontin	Noroxin	
Neutra-Phos K	K-Phos Neutral	
Norcuron	Narcan	
Noroxin	Neurontin	

Table B.1 Look-Alike and Sound-Alike Medications—*continued*

Norvasc	Navane
Novolin 70/30	NovoLog Mix 70/30
NovoLog Mix 70/30	Novolin 70/30
Occlusal-HP	Ocuflox
Ocuflox	Occlusal-Hp
opium tincture	camphorated tincture of opium (paregoric)
Os-Cal	Asacol
oxycodone	OxyContin
OxyContin	MS Contin
OxyContin	oxycodone
Pamelor	Panlor DC
Panlor DC	Pamelor
Patanol	Platinol
Paxil	Taxol
Paxil	Plavix
Percocet	Procet
Pilocar	Dilacor XR
Platinol	Patanol
Plavix	Paxil
Plendil	Isordil
pneumococcal 7 valent vaccine	pneumococcal polyvalent vaccine
pneumococcal polyvalent vaccine	pneumococcal 7 valent vaccine
Prandin	Avandia
Precare	Precose
Precose	Precare
Prilosec	Prozac
probenecid	Procanbid
Procanbid	Probenecid
Procardia XL	Protain XL
Procet	Percocet
propylthiouracil	Purinethol
Protain XL	Procardia XL
protamine	Protonix
Proton Pump Inhibitors	aripiprazole
Protonix	Lotronex
Protonix	protamine
Prozac	Prilosec
Purinethol	propylthiouracil
quinine	quinidine
quinidine	quinine
rabeprazole	aripiprazole
Recombivax HB	Comvax
Regranex	Granulex
Reminyl	Robinul
Reminyl	Amaryl
Retrovir	ritonavir
Rifadin	Rifater

Continues

Table B.1 Look-Alike and Sound-Alike Medications—*continued*

Rifater	Rifadin
Ritalin	ritodrine
Ritalin LA	Ritalin-SR
Ritalin-SR	Ritalin LA
ritodrine	Ritalin
ritonavir	Retrovir
rituximab	infliximab
Robinul	Reminyl
Roxanol	Roxicodone Intensol
Roxanol	Roxicet
Roxicet	Roxanol
Roxicodone Intensol	Roxanol
saquinavir (free base)	saquinavir mesylate
saquinavir mesylate	saquinavir (free base)
Saquinivir	Sinequan
Sarafem	Serophene
Serophene	Sarafem
Seroquel	Serzone
sertraline	Soriatane
Serzone	Seroquel
Sinequan	Saquinivir
Solu-Medrol	Depo-Medrol
Soriatane	sertraline
sufentanil	fentanyl
sumatriptan	zolmitriptan
Taxol	Taxotere
Taxol	Paxil
Taxotere	Taxol
Tegretol	Tequin
Tegretol	Tegretol XR
Tegretol XR	Tegretol
Tequin	Tegretol
Tequin	Ticlid
Testoderm	Testoderm w/Adhesive
Testoderm w/ Adhesive	Testoderm
tetanus diptheria toxoid (Td)	tuberculin purified protein derivative (PPD)
tiagabine	tizanidine
Tiazac	Ziac
Ticlid	Tequin
tizanidine	tiagabine
TNKase	Activase
TNKase	t-PA
Tobradex	Tobrex
Tobrex	TobraDex
Topamax	Toprol-XL
Toprol-XL	Topamax
Toradol	Foradil
t-PA	TNKase
Tracleer	TriCor

Table B.1 Look-Alike and Sound-Alike Medications—*continued*

tramadol hydrochloride	trazodone hydrochloride
trazodone hydrochloride	tramadol hydrochloride
tretinoin	isotretinoin
TriCor	Tracleer
tuberculin purified protein derivative (PPD)	tetanus diptheria toxoid (Td)
Tylenol	Tylenol PM
Tylenol PM	Tylenol
Ultracet	Duricef
valacyclovir	valganciclovir
Valcyte	Valtrex
valganciclovir	valacyclovir
Valtrex	Valcyte
Varivax	VZIG
Vexol	VōSol
Viagra	Allegra
vinblastine	vincristine
vincristine	vinblastine
Viokase	Viokase 8
Viokase 8	Viokase
Viracept	Viramune
Viramune	Viracept
VōSol	Vexol
VZIG	Varivax
Wellbutrin SR	Wellbutrin XL
Wellbutrin XL	Wellbutrin SR
Xeloda	Xenical
Xenical	Xeloda
Zantac	Zyrtec
Zebeta	DiaBeta
Zebeta	Zetia
Zestril	Zetia
Zetia	Zebeta
Zetia	Zestril
Ziac	Tiazac
Zocor	Cozaar
zolmitriptan	sumatriptan
Zostrix	Zovirax
Zovirax	Zyvox
Zovirax	Zostrix
Zyban	Diovan
Zyprexa	Zyrtec
Zyprexa	Celexa
Zyrtec	Zyprexa
Zyrtec	Zantac
Zyrtec	Lipitor
Zyvox	Zovirax

Source: This information was reported in the ISMP Medication Safety Alert! AcuteCare Edition, January 1996-September 2004. © 2005 Institute for Safe Medication Practices. This material is used with permission of ISMP.

Measures and Conversions

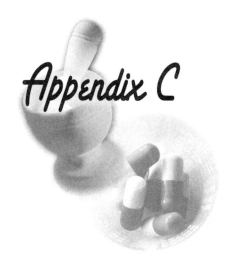

Appendix C

Metric

Volume
1 L = 1000 mL
1 mL = 1 cc
Weight
1 g = 1000 mg
1 mg = 1000 mcg

Household

Volume
1 gallon = 4 quarts
1 qt = 2 pt
1 pt = 2 cups = 16 fl oz
1 fl oz = 2 tbsp = 6 tsp
Weight
1 lb = 16 oz
Length
1 yard = 3 feet
1 foot = 12 inches

Conversions

	Household	Apothecary	Metric
Volume	1 qt = 32 fl oz		0.96 L
	1 pint = 16 fl oz		480 mL*
	1 cup = 8 fl oz		240 mL
	2 tbsp = 1 fl oz	6 fluidrams = 1 fluidounce	30 mL*
	1 tbsp	3 fluidrams	15 mL
	1 tsp	1 fluidram	5 mL**
		1 minim	0.0625 mL
Weight	2.2 lb		1 kg
	1 lb		454 g
	1 oz	8 drams	30 g
Length	1 inch		2.5 cm

* There are actually less than 30 mL in 1 fl oz, but 30 mL is usually used. When packaging a pint, companies will typically include 473 mL, rather than the full 480 mL, thus saving money over time.

** There are actually 3.75 mL in an apothecary fluidram. However, convention dictates that 1 fluidram = 5 mL = 1 tsp.

Reading Drug Labels

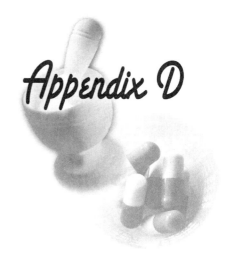

Appendix D

Figure D.1 identifies the standard parts of a drug label. The label of a brand name drug will indicate both the trade and generic names. Medications with a given name (brand or generic) are frequently available in a variety of strengths, doses, or dose forms, and information about the particular strength, dose, and dose form is also clearly stated on the drug label. Digoxin, for instance, is available as a generic product and as several branded preparations. It is available as a tablet in two different strengths (0.125 mg and 0.25 mg), a capsule in three strengths (0.05 mg, 0.1 mg, and 0.2 mg), an elixir of 0.05 mg/mL, and injections of 0.1 mg/mL and 0.25 mg/mL. Many other drugs present a similar array of choices (brand names, dosage forms, strengths, or concentrations), and the proper product to select must be made clear in the prescription order.

Figure D.1

Parts of a Drug Label

(a) brand name,
(b) generic name,
(c) dose form,
(d) strength per unit,
(e) package size,
(f) manufacturer,
(g) National Drug Code (NDC),
(h) special storage and handling requirements
(Reproduced with permission from Pfizer, Inc. All rights reserved.)

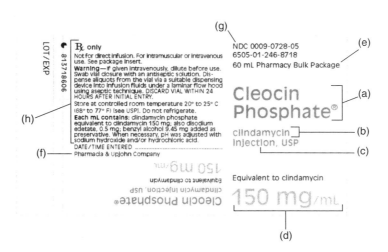

Most Commonly Prescribed Drugs

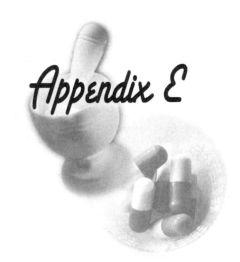

Appendix E

Generic Name	Pronunciation	Category	Brand Name
acetaminophen-codeine	a-seat-a-MIN-oh-fen KOE-deen	analgesic	Phenaphen with Codeine
acetaminophen-codeine	a-seat-a-MIN-oh-fen KOE-deen	analgesic	Tylenol with Codeine
albuterol	al-BYOO-ter-ole	bronchodilator	Proventil
albuterol	al-BYOO-ter-ole	bronchodilator	Ventolin
alendronate	a-LEN-droe-nate	bone resorption inhibitor	Fosamax
allopurinol	al-oh-PURE-i-nole	antigout agent	Zyloprim
alprazolam	al-PRAZ-oh-lam	antianxiety agent	Xanax
amitriptyline	a-mee-TRIP-ti-leen	antidepressant	Elavil
amlodipine	am-LOE-di-peen	antihypertensive	Norvasc
amlodipine-benazepril	am-LOE-di-peen ben-AYE-ze-pril	antihypertensive	Lotrel
amoxicillin	a-mox-i-SIL-in	systemic antibacterial	Trimox
amoxicillin-clavulanate	a-mox-i-SIL-in klav-yoo-LAN-ate	systemic antibacterial	Augmentin
atenolol	a-TEN-oh-lole	antihypertensive	Tenormin
atomoxetine	AT-oh-mox-e-teen	ADHD therapy agent	Strattera

Continues

Generic Name	Pronunciation	Category	Brand Name
atorvastatin	a-TOR-va-sta-tin	antihyperlipidemic	Lipitor
azithromycin	az-ith-roe-MYE-sin	systemic antibacterial	Zithromax
benazepril	ben-AYE-ze-pril	antihypertensive	Lotensin
brimonidine	bri-MOE-ni-deen	antiglaucoma agent	Alphagan P
budesonide	byoo-DES-oh-nide	antiasthmatic	Pulmicort
bupropion	byoo-PROE-pee-on	antidepressant, smoking cessation adjunct	Wellbutrin
bupropion	byoo-PROE-pee-on	antidepressant, smoking cessation adjunct	Zyban
calcitonin-salmon	kal-si-TOE-nin SAM-en	bone resorption inhibitor	Miacalcin
candesartan	kan-de-SAR-tan	antihypertensive	Atacand
carisoprodol	kar-eye-soe-PROE-dole	skeletal muscle relaxant	Soma
carvedilol	KAR-ve-dil-ole	antihypertensive	Coreg
cefdinir	sef-DI-neer	systemic antibacterial	Omnicef
cefprozil	sef-PROE-zil	systemic antibacterial	Cefzil
celecoxib	sel-a-KOX-ib	analgesic, antirheumatic NSAID	Celebrex
cephalexin	sef-a-LEX-in	systemic antibacterial	Keflex
cetirizine	se-TI-ra-zeen	antihistaminic, H_1 receptor	Zyrtec
cetirizine-pseudoephedrine	se-TI-ra-zeen soo-doe-e-FED-rin	antihistaminic, H_1 receptor–decongestant	Zyrtec-D
ciprofloxacin	sip-roe-FLOX-a-sin	systemic antibacterial	Cipro
citalopram	sye-TAL-oh-pram	antidepressant	Celexa
clarithromycin	kla-RITH-roe-mye-sin	systemic antibacterial, antimycobacterial	Biaxin
clonazepam	kloe-NA-ze-pam	anticonvulsant	Klonopin
clonidine	KLON-i-deen	antihypertensive	Catapres
clonidine	KLON-i-deen	antihypertensive	Duraclon
clopidogrel	kloh-PID-oh-grel	antithrombotic, platelet aggregation inhibitor	Plavix

Generic Name	Pronunciation	Category	Brand Name
clotrimazole-betamethasone	kloe-TRIM-a-zole bay-ta-METH-a-sone	antifungal, corticosteroid	Lotrisone
conjugated estrogen	CON-ju-gate-ed ES-troe-jen	antineoplastic, systemic estrogen, osteoporosis prophylactic, ovarian hormone therapy agent	Premarin
conjugated estrogen–medroxyprogesterone	CON-ju-gate-ed ES-troe-jen me-DROX-ee-proe-JES-te-rone	estrogen-progestin, osteoporosis prophylactic, ovarian hormone therapy agent	Premphase
conjugated estrogen–medroxyprogesterone	CON-ju-gate-ed ES-troe-jen me-DROX-ee-proe-JES-te-rone	estrogen-progestin, osteoporosis prophylactic, ovarian hormone therapy agent	Prempro
cyclobenzaprine	sye-kloe-BEN-za-preen	skeletal muscle relaxant	Flexeril
desloratadine	des-LOR-at-a-deen	antihistaminic, H$_1$ receptor	Clarinex
dextroamphetamine-amphetamine	dex-troe-am-FET-a-meen am-FET-a-meen	CNS stimulant, ADHD therapy	Adderall
diazepam	dye-AZ-e-pam	amnestic, antianxiety agent, anticonvulsant, antipanic agent, antitremor agent, sedative-hypnotic, skeletal muscle relaxant adjunct	Valium
digoxin	di-JOX-in	antiarrhythmic, cardiotonic	Lanoxicaps
digoxin	di-JOX-in	antiarrhythmic, cardiotonic	Lanoxin
diltiazem	dil-TYE-a-zem	antianginal, antiarrhythmic, antihypertensive	Cardizem
diltiazem	dil-TYE-a-zem	antianginal, antiarrhythmic, antihypertensive	Dilacor
divalproex	dye-VAL-pro-ex	anticonvulsant, antimanic, migraine headache prophylactic	Depakote
donepezil	don-EH-pa-zil	dementia symptoms treatment adjunct	Aricept
doxycycline	dox-i-SYE-kleen	systemic antibacterial, antiprotozoal	Vibramycin

Continues

Generic Name	Pronunciation	Category	Brand Name
enalapril	e-NAL-a-pril	antihypertensive, vasodilator	Vasotec
escitalopram	es-sye-TAL-oh-pram	antianxiety agent, antidepressant	Lexapro
esomeprazole	es-oh-ME-pray-zole	gastric acid pump inhibitor, antiulcer agent	Nexium
ethinyl estradiol–desogestrel	ETH-in-il es-tra-DYE-ole des-oh-JES-trel	antiendometriotic, systemic contraceptive, gonadotropin inhibitor	Cyclessa
ethinyl estradiol–desogestrel	ETH-in-il es-tra-DYE-ole des-oh-JES-trel	antiendometriotic, systemic contraceptive, gonadotropin inhibitor	Desogen
ethinyl estradiol–desogestrel	ETH-in-il es-tra-DYE-ole des-oh-JES-trel	antiendometriotic, systemic contraceptive, gonadotropin inhibitor	Kariva
ethinyl estradiol–desogestrel	ETH-in-il es-tra-DYE-ole des-oh-JES-trel	antiendometriotic, systemic contraceptive, gonadotropin inhibitor	Mircette
ethinyl estradiol–desogestrel	ETH-in-il es-tra-DYE-ole des-oh-JES-trel	antiendometriotic, systemic contraceptive, gonadotropin inhibitor	Ortho-Cept
ethinyl estradiol–drospirenone	ETH-in-il es-tra-DYE-ole droh-SPYE-re-none	systemic contraceptive	Yasmin
ethinyl estradiol–levonorgestrel	ETH-in-il es-tra-DYE-ole LEE-voe-nor-jes-trel	antiendometriotic, systemic postcoital contraceptive, systemic contraceptive, estrogen progestin, gonadotropin inhibitor	Levlen
ethinyl estradiol–levonorgestrel	ETH-in-il es-tra-DYE-ole LEE-voe-nor-jes-trel	antiendometriotic, systemic postcoital contraceptive, systemic contraceptive, estrogen progestin, gonadotropin inhibitor	Nordette
ethinyl estradiol–levonorgestrel	ETH-in-il es-tra-DYE-ole LEE-voe-nor-jes-trel	antiendometriotic, systemic postcoital contraceptive, systemic contraceptive, estrogen progestin, gonadotropin inhibitor	Seasonale

Generic Name	Pronunciation	Category	Brand Name
ethinyl estradiol–levonorgestrel	ETH-in-il es-tra-DYE-ole LEE-voe-nor-jes-trel	antiendometriotic, systemic postcoital contraceptive, systemic contraceptive, estrogen progestin, gonadotropin inhibitor	Tri-Levlen
ethinyl estradiol–levonorgestrel	ETH-in-il es-tra-DYE-ole LEE-voe-nor-jes-trel	antiendometriotic, systemic postcoital contraceptive, systemic contraceptive, estrogen progestin, gonadotropin inhibitor	Triphasil
ethinyl estradiol–levonorgestrel	ETH-in-il es-tra-DYE-ole LEE-voe-nor-jes-trel	antiendometriotic, systemic postcoital contraceptive, systemic contraceptive, estrogen progestin, gonadotropin inhibitor	Trivora-28
ethinyl estradiol–norelgestromin	ETH-in-il es-tra-DYE-ole nor-el-JES-troe-min	systemic contraceptive	Ortho Evra
ethinyl estradiol–norethindrone	ETH-in-il es-tra-DYE-ole nor-eth-IN-drone	antiacne agent, anti-endometriotic, systemic contraceptive, estrogen progestin, gonadotropin inhibitor	Estrostep Fe
ethinyl estradiol–norethindrone	ETH-in-il es-tra-DYE-ole nor-eth-IN-drone	antiacne agent, anti-endometriotic, systemic contraceptive, estrogen progestin, gonadotropin inhibitor	Femhrt
ethinyl estradiol–norethindrone	ETH-in-il es-tra-DYE-ole nor-eth-IN-drone	antiacne agent, anti-endometriotic, systemic contraceptive, estrogen progestin, gonadotropin inhibitor	Loestrin Fe
ethinyl estradiol–norethindrone	ETH-in-il es-tra-DYE-ole nor-eth-IN-drone	antiacne agent, anti-endometriotic, systemic contraceptive, estrogen progestin, gonadotropin inhibitor	Ovcon

Continues

Generic Name	Pronunciation	Category	Brand Name
ethinyl estradiol–norgestimate	ETH-in-il es-tra-DYE-ole nor-JES-ti-mate	antiacne agent, anti-endometriotic, systemic contraceptive, estrogen progestin, gonadotropin inhibitor	Ortho Tri-Cyclen
ethinyl estradiol–norgestimate	ETH-in-il es-tra-DYE-ole nor-JES-ti-mate	antiacne agent, anti-endometriotic, systemic contraceptive, estrogen progestin, gonadotropin inhibitor	Ortho Tri-Cyclen Lo
ethinyl estradiol–norgestrel	ETH-in-il es-tra-DYE-ole nor-JES-trel	antiendometriotic, systemic postcoital contraceptive, systemic contraceptive, estrogen progestin, gonadotropin inhibitor	Lo/Ovral
ethinyl estradiol–norgestrel	ETH-in-il es-tra-DYE-ole nor-JES-trel	antiendometriotic, systemic postcoital contraceptive, systemic contraceptive, estrogen progestin, gonadotropin inhibitor	Low-Ogestrel
ethinyl estradiol–norgestrel	ETH-in-il es-tra-DYE-ole nor-JES-trel	antiendometriotic, systemic postcoital contraceptive, systemic contraceptive, estrogen progestin, gonadotropin inhibitor	Ovral
ezetimibe	e-ZET-e-mibe	antihyperlipidemic	Zetia
felodipine	fe-LOE-di-peen	antianginal, antihypertensive	Plendil
fenofibrate	fen-oh-FYE-brate	antihyperlipidemic	Tricor
fentanyl	FEN-ta-nil	analgesic, anesthesia adjunct	Actiq
fentanyl	FEN-ta-nil	analgesic	Duragesic
fentanyl	FEN-ta-nil	analgesic, anesthesia adjunct	Sublimaze
fexofenadine	fex-o-FEN-a-deen	antihistaminic, H_1 receptor	Allegra
fexofenadine-pseudoephedrine	fex-o-FEN-a-deen soo-doe-e-FED-rin	antihistaminic, H_1 receptor–decongestant	Allegra-D

Generic Name	Pronunciation	Category	Brand Name
finasteride	fin-AS-tur-ide	benign prostatic hyper-plasia therapy agent, hair growth stimulant	Propecia
finasteride	fin-AS-tur-ide	benign prostatic hyper-plasia therapy agent, hair growth stimulant	Proscar
fluconazole	floo-KOE-na-zole	systemic antifungal	Diflucan
fluoxetine	floo-OX-e-teen	antidepressant, anti-obsessional agent, antibulemic agent	Prozac
fluoxetine	floo-OX-e-teen	antidepressant, anti-obsessional agent, antibulemic agent	Sarafem
fluticasone	floo-TIK-a-sone	steroidal nasal anti-inflammatory, nasal corticosteroid	Flonase
fluticasone	floo-TIK-a-sone	steroidal nasal anti-inflammatory, nasal corticosteroid	Flovent
fluticasone-salmeterol	floo-TIK-a-sone sal-ME-te-role	antiasthmatic, inhalation antiinflammatory, bronchodilator	Advair Diskus
fluvastatin	FLOO-va-sta-tin	antihyperlipidemic, HMG-CoA reductase inhibitor	Lescol
folic acid	FOE-lik AS-id	diagnostic aid, folate deficiency, nutritional vitamin supplement	many
fosinopril	foe-SIN-oh-pril	antihypertensive, vasodilator	Monopril
furosemide	fur-OH-se-mide	antihypercalcemic, antihypertensive, renal disease diagnostic aid adjunct, diuretic	Lasix
gabapentin	GA-ba-pen-tin	anticonvulsant, antineuralgic	Neurontin
gemfibrozil	jem-FI-broe-zil	antihyperlipidimic	Lopid
glimepiride	GLYE-me-pye-ride	antidiabetic	Amaryl

Continues

Generic Name	Pronunciation	Category	Brand Name
glipizide	GLIP-i-zide	antidiabetic	Glucotrol
glyburide	GLYE-byoo-ride	antidiabetic	DiaBeta
glyburide	GLYE-byoo-ride	antidiabetic	Glynase
glyburide	GLYE-byoo-ride	antidiabetic	Micronase
glyburide-metformin	GLYE-byoo-ride met-FOR-min	antidiabetic	Glucovance
hydrochlorothiazide	hye-droe-klor-oh-THYE-a-zide	antihypertensive, diuretic, antiurolithic	Esidrix
hydrocodone-acetaminophen	hye-droe-KOE-done a-seat-a-MIN-oh-fen	analgesic	Lortab
hydrocodone-acetaminophen	hye-droe-KOE-done a-seat-a-MIN-oh-fen	analgesic	Vicodin
hydrocodone-chlorpheniramine	hye-droe-KOE-done klor-fen-EER-a-meen	antihistaminic, H_1 receptor–antitussive	Tussionex
ibuprofen	eye-byoo-PROE-fen	analgesic	Advil
ibuprofen	eye-byoo-PROE-fen	analgesic	Motrin
insulin glargine	IN-su-lin GLARE-jeen	antidiabetic	Lantus
insulin lispro	IN-su-lin LYE-sproe	antidiabetic	Humalog
ipratropium	i-pra-TROE-pee-um	antiasthmatic	Atrovent
ipratropium-albuterol	i-pra-TROE-pee-um al-BYOO-ter-ole	antiasthmatic-bronchodilator	Combivent
irbesartan	ir-be-SAR-tan	antihypertensive	Avapro
irbesartan-hydrochlorothiazide	ir-be-SAR-tan hye-droe-klor-oh-THYE-a-zide	antihypertensive, diuretic	Avalide
isosorbide mononitrate	eye-soe-SOR-bide mon-oh-NYE-trate	antianginal	Imdur
isosorbide mononitrate	eye-soe-SOR-bide mon-oh-NYE-trate	antianginal	Ismo
lansoprazole	lan-SOE-pra-zole	gastric acid pump inhibitor, antiulcer agent	Prevacid
latanoprost	la-TA-noe-prost	antiglaucoma agent, ocular antihypertensive	Xalatan

Generic Name	Pronunciation	Category	Brand Name
levofloxacin	lee-voe-FLOX-a-sin	systemic antibacterial	Levaquin
levothyroxine, T_4	lee-voe-thye-ROX-een	antineoplastic, thyroid function diagnostic aid, thyroid hormone	Levothroid
levothyroxine, T_4	lee-voe-thye-ROX-een	antineoplastic, thyroid function diagnostic aid, thyroid hormone	Synthroid
lisinopril	lyse-IN-oh-pril	antihypertensive, vasodilator	Prinivil
lisinopril	lyse-IN-oh-pril	antihypertensive, vasodilator	Zestril
lorazepam	lor-AZ-e-pam	amnestic, antianxiety agent, anticonvulsant, antiemetic, antipanic agent, antitremor agent, sedative-hypnotic, skeletal muscle relaxant	Ativan
losartan	loe-SAR-tan	angiotensin II–receptor antagonist, antihypertensive	Cozaar
losartan-hydrochlorothiazide	loe-SAR-tan hye-droe-klor-oh-THYE-a-zide	antihypertensive	Hyzaar
meclizine	MEK-li-zeen	antiemetic, antivertigo agent	Antivert
meloxicam	mel-OX-i-kam	antirheumatic (NSAID)	Mobic
metaxalone	me-TAX-a-lone	skeletal muscle relaxant	Skelaxin
metformin	met-FOR-min	antihyperglycemic	Glucophage
methylphenidate	meth-il-FEN-i-date	CNS stimulant, ADHD therapy	Concerta
methylphenidate	meth-il-FEN-i-date	CNS stimulant, ADHD therapy	Metadate
methylphenidate	meth-il-FEN-i-date	CNS stimulant, ADHD therapy	Ritalin
methylprednisolone	meth-il-pred-NIS-oh-lone	steroidal antiinflammatory, corticoid steroid, immunosuppressant	Medrol

Continues

Generic Name	Pronunciation	Category	Brand Name
metoprolol	met-oh-PROE-lole	antiadrenergic, antianginal, antianxiety therapy adjunct, antiarrhythmic, antihypertensive, antitremor agent, hypertrophic cardiomyopathy therapy adjunct, myocardial infarction therapy, neuroleptic-induced akathisia therapy, pheochromocytoma therapy adjunct, thyrotoxicosis therapy adjunct, vascular headache prophylactic	Lopressor
metoprolol	met-oh-PROE-lole	antiadrenergic, antianginal, antianxiety therapy adjunct, antiarrhythmic, antihypertensive, antitremor agent, hypertrophic cardiomyopathy therapy adjunct, myocardial infarction therapy, neuroleptic-induced akathisia therapy, pheochromocytoma therapy adjunct, thyrotoxicosis therapy adjunct, vascular headache prophylactic	Toprol
mirtazapine	mir-TAZ-a-peen	antidepressant	Remeron
mometasone furoate	moe-MET-a-sone FYOOR-oh-ate	nasal steroidal anti-inflammatory, nasal corticosteroid	Nasonex
montelukast	mon-te-LOO-kast	antiasthmatic, leukotriene receptor antagonist	Singulair
moxifloxacin	mox-i-FLOX-a-sin	systemic antibacterial	Avelox
moxifloxacin	mox-i-FLOX-a-sin	ophthalmic antibacterial	Vigamox
mupirocin	myoo-PEER-oh-sin	topical antibacterial	Bactroban
naproxen	na-PROX-en	analgesic, nonsteroidal antiinflammatory, antidysmenorrheal, antigout agent, antipyretic, nonsteroidal antiinflammatory antirheumatic, vascular headache prophylactic, vascular headache suppressant	Aleve

Generic Name	Pronunciation	Category	Brand Name
naproxen	na-PROX-en	analgesic, nonsteroidal antiinflammatory, antidysmenorrheal, antigout agent, antipyretic, nonsteroidal antiinflammatory antirheumatic, vascular headache prophylactic, vascular headache suppressant	Naprosyn
niacin	NYE-a-sin	nutritional supplement, vitamin	Niacor
nifedipine	nye-FED-i-peen	antianginal, antihypertensive	Procardia
nitrofurantoin	nye-troe-fyoor-AN-toyn	systemic antibacterial	Macrobid
nitrofurantoin	nye-troe-fyoor-AN-toyn	systemic antibacterial	Macrodantin
nitroglycerin	nye-troe-GLI-ser-in	antianginal, congestive heart failure vasodilator	Minitran
nitroglycerin	nye-troe-GLI-ser-in	antianginal, congestive heart failure vasodilator	Nitrolingual
nitroglycerin	nye-troe-GLI-ser-in	antianginal, congestive heart failure vasodilator	Nitrostat
NPH isophane insulin	NPH EYE-so-fayn IN-su-lin	antidiabetic	Humulin N
NPH regular insulin	NPH REG-u-lar IN-su-lin	antidiabetic	Humulin 70/30
olanzapine	oh-LAN-za-peen	antipsychotic	Zyprexa
olopatadine	oh-loe-pa-TA-deen	ophthalmic antihistaminic, H_1 receptor; ophthalmic mast cell stabilizer; ophthalmic antiallergic	Patanol
omeprazole	oh-ME-pray-zole	gastric acid pump inhibitor, antiulcer agent	Prilosec
oxybutynin	ox-i-BYOO-ti-nin	urinary tract antispasmodic	Ditropan
oxycodone	ox-i-KOE-done	analgesic	OxyContin
oxycodone-acetaminophen	ox-i-KOE-done a-seat-a-MIN-oh-fen	analgesic	Endocet
oxycodone-acetaminophen	ox-i-KOE-done a-seat-a-MIN-oh-fen	analgesic	Percocet

Continues

Generic Name	Pronunciation	Category	Brand Name
oxycodone-acetaminophen	ox-i-KOE-done a-seat-a-MIN-oh-fen	analgesic	Tylox
pantoprazole	pan-TOE-pray-zole	gastric acid pump inhibitor, antiulcer agent	Protonix
paroxetine	pa-ROX-e-teen	antianxiety agent, antidepressant, antiobsessional agent, antipanic agent, posttraumatic stress disorder agent, social anxiety disorder agent	Paxil
penicillin V	pen-i-SIL-in V	systemic antibacterial	Veetids
phenytoin	FEN-i-toyn	antiarrhythmic, anticonvulsant, trigeminal neuralgic antineuralgic, skeletal muscle relaxant	Dilantin
pimecrolimus	pim-e-KROW-li-mus	immunomodulator	Elidel
pioglitazone	pye-oh-GLI-ta-zone	antidiabetic	Actos
polyethylene glycol	pol-ee-ETH-il-een GLYE-kole	hyperosmotic laxative	Miralax
potassium chloride	poe-tass-EE-um KLOR-ide	antihypokalemic, electrolyte replenisher	Klor-Con
pravastatin	PRA-va-sta-tin	antihyperlipidemic, HMG-CoA reductase inhibitor	Pravachol
prednisone	PRED-ni-sone	steroidal inflammatory, cancer chemotherapy antiemetic, corticosteroid, immunosuppressant	Deltasone
promethazine	proe-METH-a-zeen	antiemetic; antihistaminic, H_1 receptor; antivertigo agent; sedative-hypnotic	Phenergan
promethazine-codeine	proe-METH-a-zeen KOE-deen	antihistaminic, H_1 receptor-antitussive	Promethazine with Codeine
propoxyphene-acetaminophen	proe-POX-i-feen a-seat-a-MIN-oh-fen	analgesic	Darvocet-N 100

Generic Name	Pronunciation	Category	Brand Name
propranolol	proe-PRAN-oh-lole	antiadrenergic, antianginal, antianxiety therapy adjunct, antiarrhythmic, antihypertensive, antitremor agent, hypertrophic cardiomyopathy therapy adjunct, myocardial infarction prophylactic, myocardial infarction therapy, neuroleptic-induced akathisia therapy, pheochromocytoma therapy adjunct, thyrotoxicosis therapy adjunct, vascular headache prophylactic	Inderal
quetiapine	kwe-TYE-a-peen	antipsychotic	Seroquel
quinapril	KWIN-a-pril	antihypertensive, vasodilator	Accupril
rabeprazole	ra-BE-pray-zole	gastric acid pump inhibitor, antiulcer agent	Aciphex
raloxifene	ral-OX-i-feen	selective estrogen receptor modulator, osteoporosis prophylactic	Evista
ramipril	RA-mi-pril	antihypertensive, vasodilator	Altace
ranitidine	ra-NI-ti-deen	histamine H_2–receptor antagonist, antiulcer agent, gastric acid secretion inhibitor	Zantac
risedronate	ris-ED-roe-nate	bone resorption inhibitor	Actonel
risperidone	ris-PER-i-done	antipsychotic	Risperdal
rosiglitazone	ROS-e-glit-a-zone	antidiabetic	Avandia
sertraline	SER-tra-leen	antianxiety agent, antidepressant, antiobsessional agent, antipanic agent, posttraumatic stress disorder therapy agent, premenstrual dysphoric disorder therapy agent	Zoloft

Continues

Most Commonly Prescribed Drugs • *Appendix E*   **139**

Generic Name	Pronunciation	Category	Brand Name
sildenafil	sil-DEN-a-fil	systemic impotence therapy agent	Viagra
simvastatin	SIM-va-sta-tin	antihyperlipidemic, HMG-CoA reductase inhibitor	Zocor
spironolactone	speer-on-oh-LAK-tone	aldosterone antagonist, antihypertensive, antihy-pokalemic, primary hyper-aldosteronism diagnostic aid, diuretic	Aldactone
sulfamethoxazole-trimethoprim	sul-fa-meth-OX-a-zole trye-METH-oh-prim	systemic antibacterial, antiprotozoal	Bactrim
sulfamethoxazole-trimethoprim	sul-fa-meth-OX-a-zole trye-METH-oh-prim	systemic antibacterial, antiprotozoal	Cotrim
sulfamethoxazole-trimethoprim	sul-fa-meth-OX-a-zole trye-METH-oh-prim	systemic antibacterial, antiprotozoal	Septra DS
sumatriptan	soo-ma-TRIP-tan	antimigraine agent	Imitrex
tamsulosin	tam-SOO-loh-sin	benign prostatic hyper plasia therapy agent	Flomax
temazepam	tem-AZ-e-pam	sedative-hypnotic	Restoril
terazosin	ter-AYE-zoe-sin	antihypertensive, benign prostatic hyperplasia therapy agent	Hytrin
timolol	TYE-moe-lole	antiadrenergic, antianginal, antianxiety therapy adjunct, antiarrhythmic, systemic antiglaucoma agent, antihypertensive, antitremor agent, hyper-trophic cardiomyopathy therapy adjunct, myocar-dial infarction prophylactic, pheochromocytoma therapy adjunct, thyro-toxicosis therapy adjunct, vascular headache prophylactic	Blocadren
timolol	TYE-moe-lole	ophthalmic antiglaucoma agent	Timoptic

Generic Name	Pronunciation	Category	Brand Name
tobramycin-dexamethasone	toe-bra-MYE-sin dex-a-METH-a-sone	ophthalmic corticosteroid, ophthalmic steroidal anti-inflammatory, ophthalmic antibacterial	TobraDex
tolterodine	TOLE-tear-oh-deen	urinary bladder antispasmodic	Detrol
topiramate	toe-PYRE-a-mate	anticonvulsant, anti-migraine headache	Topamax
tramadol	TRA-ma-dole	analgesic	Ultram
tramadol-acetaminophen	TRA-ma-dole a-seat-a-MIN-oh-fen	analgesic	Ultracet
trazodone	TRAZ-oh-done	antidepressant, antineuralgic	Desyrel
triamcinolone	trye-am-SIN-oh-lone	inhalation anti-inflammatory, antiasthmatic	Azmacort
triamcinolone	trye-am-SIN-oh-lone	nasal steroidal anti-inflammatory, nasal corticosteroid	Nasacort AQ
triamterene-hydrochlorothiazide	trye-AM-ter-een hye-droe-klor-oh-THYE-a-zide	antihypertensive, antihypokalemic, diuretic	Dyazide
triamterene-hydrochlorothiazide	trye-AM-ter-een hye-droe-klor-oh-THYE-a-zide	antihypertensive, antihypokalemic, diuretic	Maxzide
valacyclovir	val-ay-SYE-kloe-veer	systemic antiviral	Valtrex
valsartan	val-SAR-tan	antihypertensive	Diovan
valsartan-hydrochlorothiazide	val-SAR-tan hye-droe-klor-oh-THYE-a-zide	antihypertensive	Diovan HCT
venlafaxine	ven-la-FAX-een	antidepressant, antianxiety agent	Effexor
verapamil	ver-AP-a-mil	antianginal, antiarrhythmic, antihypertensive, hypertrophic cardiomyopathy therapy adjunct, vascular headache prophylactic	Calan

Continues

Generic Name	Pronunciation	Category	Brand Name
verapamil	ver-AP-a-mil	antianginal, antiarrhythmic, antihypertensive, hypertrophic cardiomyopathy therapy adjunct, vascular headache prophylactic	Covera HS
verapamil	ver-AP-a-mil	antianginal, antiarrhythmic, antihypertensive, hypertrophic cardiomyopathy therapy adjunct, vascular headache prophylactic	Isoptin
verapamil	ver-AP-a-mil	antianginal, antiarrhythmic, antihypertensive, hypertrophic cardiomyopathy therapy adjunct, vascular headache prophylactic	Verelan
warfarin	WAR-far-in	anticoagulant	Coumadin
zolpidem	ZOLE-pi-dem	sedative hypnotic	Ambien

SOURCE: Adapted from RxList, The Top 200 Prescriptions for 2003 by Number of U.S. Prescriptions Dispensed: Generic Name (http://www.rxlist.com/top200.htm, accessed 8-24-2004). Category information from the U.S. National Library of Medicine and National Institutes of Health MedlinePlus Web site (http://www.nlm.nih.gov/medlineplus/, accessed 12-17-2004).